Doing
the
Right
Thing

An Approach to
Moral Issues in
Mental Health
Treatment

Doing the Right Thing

*An Approach to
Moral Issues in
Mental Health
Treatment*

John R. Peteet, M.D.

*Associate Professor of Psychiatry
Harvard Medical School
Brigham and Women's Hospital
Dana-Farber Cancer Institute
Boston, Massachusetts*

American
Psychiatric
Publishing, Inc.

Washington, DC
London, England

Manufactured in the United States of America on acid-free paper
08 07 06 05 04   5 4 3 2 1
First Edition

Typeset in Palatino, Formata, and Galahad

American Psychiatric Publishing, Inc.
1000 Wilson Boulevard
Arlington, VA 22209–3901
www.appi.org

Library of Congress Cataloging-in-Publication Data
Peteet, John R., 1947–
    Doing the right thing : an approach to moral issues in mental health
treatment / John R. Peteet
        p. ; cm.
    Includes bibliographical references and index.
    ISBN 1-58562-083-1 (alk. paper)
    1. Psychotherapy—Moral and ethical aspects. I. Title.
    [DNLM: 1. Psychotherapy—ethics. 2. Moral Obligations.
WM420 P4775d 2004]
    RC455.2.E8P467 2004
    174.2—dc22

                                                            2003058306

British Library Cataloguing in Publication Data
A CIP record is available from the British Library.

Contents

Introduction

> There is only one duty, only one safe course, and
> that is to try to be right.
>
> *Winston Churchill*

An engaging woman in her mid-20s saw me because of anxiety, sleeplessness, and irritability. She had been preoccupied with helping her husband stop drinking and with deciding how to respond to her brother's requests that she cover for his shady business practices. Having recently read *Codependent No More,* she wondered if she felt overly responsible for others' problems.

We began to explore the basis of her standards. To what extent did she feel obligated to help others even at her own expense? How had her view of herself as the family caretaker developed? How did she understand and weigh her responsibilities toward her husband, her brother, and herself? It soon became evident that she had played the role of mediator since before her parents' divorce 10 years earlier and that a desire to help family members remained an important part of her identity.

Talking helped her to clarify how her conscience had developed, but I wondered: Was it also my task to help her change the way it worked? For example, should I encourage her to reassess her standards and modify her goals so as to make them more achievable, or "realistic"?

A successful salesman in his early 50s reluctantly agreed to see a psychiatrist after his wife of 26 years threatened to leave because of his intermittently sarcastic and verbally abusive behavior. He described himself as "not proud of behaving like a jerk at times," but his psychiatrist wondered whether he was distressed enough to work at saving his marriage.

Should a therapist confront not only this patient's denial but also his lack of empathy and his limited capacity for experiencing guilt? If as a result of treatment the patient felt more appropriately guilty, how should his therapist help him to deal with this? What psychotherapeutic paradigm should he follow?

Many other situations familiar to clinicians raise questions about their role in patients' moral lives. How can therapists help individuals struggling with whether it is right for them to divorce, if and how to forgive a childhood abuser, or how much to sacrifice for an aging parent? How should they respond to a patient who is harming others—for example, by engaging in unsafe sex with random partners, driving drunk, or neglecting her children? How should they deal with patients convinced that they deserve to suffer—for example, the abuse survivor whose deeply rooted sense of shame drives her to continue cutting herself? What can a therapist do to help a young cancer patient trying to understand whether fairness exists?

Mental health clinicians lack consensus on how to approach such questions. Some rely on abstract principles such as neutrality, professional codes of ethics, or legal mandates to report abuse. Others respond on the basis of their personal values. Many avoid dealing explicitly with moral issues, for several reasons: Freud recognized the importance of the superego to the psychic life but maintained, as did many of his followers (Gedo 1986; Gilligan 1976), that psychiatry's scientific, pragmatic orientation implies a "neutral" attitude toward more philosophical questions such as what is good and right (except perhaps for an assumed commitment to enhance patient autonomy). Clinicians often recognize the importance of personal values but assume that tolerance is the only basis for consensus, fearing that discussing value differences in treatment will be distracting and/or threatening to the therapeutic alliance. Working every day with patients whose neurotic guilt impedes their insight and freedom of choice can encourage therapists to associate morality with punishment and blame. Many regard individuals who focus on morality as moralistic—that is, presumptuous, judgmental, and possibly hypocritical.

This avoidance has costs. Without acknowledging that they have a moral role when they promote being fully human, mental health professionals can convey that they are indifferent to their patients' concerns about what is right, or that therapy is at least amoral, if not potentially destructive to patients' moral and spiritual values (Cushman 1995; Lomas 1999; Stone 1984). Patients sometimes need therapists to help them take their philosophies of life into account in making difficult decisions. Furthermore, therapists who do not examine their own values can remain unaware of how these commitments influence their work, just as countertransferential responses do.

The problem is not that clinicians lack personal or professional values. Therapists have long believed in respecting their patients' autonomy, and in response to the market-based priorities of managed care, they have recently articulated other shared ideals, notably the need to care for patients as human beings rather than as commodities (Pellegrino and Thomasma 1997). Professional meetings frequently have humanistic themes such as equity, equal access, high-quality care, and ending stigma. Workshops, as well as a growing literature, consider how to uphold the values of informed consent, confidentiality, respectful boundaries, and the fair allocation of scarce resources.

However, broad ethical principles such as therapeutic neutrality (Alonso 1996; Hoffer 1991) and *primum non nocere* (first do no harm) are of only limited help to clinicians in facing specific questions about their moral role in contemporary eclectic treatments that may include cognitive, behavioral, psychodynamic, and interpersonal interventions. Acting instead on the basis of their own personal values, particularly if these remain unarticulated, risks a private form of paternalism.

The purpose of this book is to offer a more adequate framework for discussing and approaching moral issues arising in treatment. The framework for this moral paradigm centers on the concept of moral functioning. Morality orients the self in relation to what is most important, guides the process of living with others in society, and encourages both self-evaluation and changes in course. To live well, individuals must be able to achieve basic moral ends—that is, develop core moral commitments, make moral decisions, implement moral plans, assess the rightness of their behavior, deal with moral failure, and develop morally admired character traits or virtues. The process of accomplishing these ends is analogous to the functioning of other systems that are basic to healthy living, including the physical (made up of sensory, reproductive, excretory, and other subsystems), emotional, and social. Moral functioning has physical, affective, and relational components but is not reducible to any of them. As a consequence, to address problems in this area, clinicians must use a moral paradigm in the same way that they use biological, intrapsychic, or relational paradigms to assess and address problems in these domains.

Incorporating a moral paradigm into mental health treatment may seem to some readers like crossing a boundary. However, psychiatry and related clinical disciplines have long shared a moral identity with medicine. Physicians are scientific in that they investigate the nature of disease, humanistic in that they investigate the experience of the patient, and moral in that they act on behalf of patients' best interests. Individual clinicians may differ in their private morality but agree on many health-related values, including self-care, respect, and responsibility. Few would dispute that good medical treatment depends on the clinician's basic moral character—that is, on humility, honesty, intellectual integrity, compassion, and effacement of excessive self-interest (Pellegrino and Thomasma 1993). Mental health treatment is also concerned with the optimal functioning of the whole person within a context of relationships and meaning. Virtues essential for psychotherapists include caring, respect, courage, and the ability to maintain professional boundaries (Doherty 1995; Will 1981).

The chapters that follow explore the implications of a functional paradigm for understanding the clinician's role in dealing with the moral aspects of several common clinical concerns: influencing patients, deciding on the direction of treatment, understanding problems in caring, approaching moral dilemmas, and dealing with unfair pain and with moral failure. The last two chapters discuss the therapeutic potential of moral growth and transformation and the possibility of achieving needed integration through the use of a moral paradigm. As the penultimate chapters more frequently ask questions and suggest possibilities than provide answers, the reader interested in a coherent statement of the book's central message may want to begin with the final chapter.

Because most readers will have a preferred way of understanding morality (about which they may feel deeply), they should try to be patient at the outset in considering whether the terminology chosen here to describe moral functioning proves useful. The term *moral* has been used in various ways, often interchangeably with the term *ethical*. By convention, the term *moral* here refers to what is good, right, or ideal (in the sense of how things ought—or ought not—to be), and *ethical* refers to the means of achieving moral ends (as in the case of the physician trying to balance his concern for the welfare of an uncooperative patient with respect for the latter's autonomy). The use of such terms that refer to what is ultimately good or ideal of course raises philosophical and spiritual questions: about whether there are moral universals and what their content might be; about whether morality depends on an external, objective, or transcendent reality; and about what that reality is. These questions are often important to patients, but my purpose here is more limited and pragmatic: 1) to understand what people need to do in order to function morally; 2) to consider, using case examples, the way in which this understanding of morality informs several of our core roles as mental health clinicians; and 3) to apply this understanding to the common moral challenges that clinicians face. Eventually, of course, adopting even a pragmatic or task-oriented view of morality will bring us to consider whether there are certain core moral values integral to healthy mental functioning (Doherty 1995; Jensen and Bergin 1988; Nicholas 1994). Agreeing on these, of course, does not mean that clinicians should try to impose them on their patients.

Chapter 1 considers what is appropriate influence on a patient by a therapist. Should therapists try to minimize the influence of their own commitments by taking a nondirective or abstinent stance? Should they focus on obtaining informed consent? assume that their influence is inevitable and expect patients to welcome it? or try to distinguish therapeutic from technical neutrality? Each of these approaches has its use, but none alone is an adequate basis for acting as a moral agent in the patient's life.

A better basis may be directly addressing problems in moral functioning. Effectively achieving moral ends requires the capacities to develop moral commitments, make and implement moral decisions, assess the rightness of their behavior, deal with moral failure, and develop morally admired character traits or virtues. What tends to interfere with the development of these capacities, and in what ways? Identifying problems in an individual's moral functioning is a first step in formulating a treatment plan that takes the therapist's moral influence into account.

Chapter 2 addresses how values held by the clinician, the patient, and/or third parties should influence the direction of treatment—for example, when a patient requests medication to relieve anxiety but his therapist believes he should bear it. Planning a treatment course in such cases becomes a process of moral reasoning: assessing the facts of the case, identifying the moral question involved, considering a full range of aims and paradigms (e.g., biological, behavioral, intrapsychic, relational, developmental, existential, and moral), and selecting paradigms by taking therapeutic and other values into account.

It also involves deciding what to actually do in the face of resistance. Resistance is sometimes cognitive, reflecting difficulty understanding the nature of the therapeutic task. For example, patients sometimes fail to comprehend how exploring the past could help relieve current symptoms. At other times resistance is primarily affective, reflecting difficulty in relinquishing long-held maladaptive patterns or bearing painful affects. Moral resistance may stem from a patient's guilt or uncertainty about what is right for him. For example, an abuse survivor may be convinced that she ought to sacrifice her needs to those of others even when the predictable outcome is that she becomes emotionally overwhelmed. To help her move forward, a therapist would assess whether there are situational or pervasive problems in her moral functioning that should themselves become a focus of the work.

Chapter 3 explores problems in caring for patients. Students of caring have traditionally used potentially complementary but poorly integrated models of caring: feeling empathy, accepting responsibility for others' welfare, nurturing patients, or attending to the details of their needs. From a moral perspective, caring is a dynamic process that involves developing and clarifying caring commitments; incorporating these commitments into one's decision making; implementing decisions in relation to competing priorities; assessing how well another person's needs are being met; correcting failures to care effectively; and finding support for caring better. Understanding this process offers specific ways to foster caring and deal adequately with clinicians who offend or harm patients.

Chapter 4 examines how patients and clinicians can best deal with moral dilemmas arising in treatment. Patients may ask, "How much should I sacrifice for my aging parent?" or "Should I get divorced?" or "Is it right for my boss to treat me this way?"—reflecting difficulties balancing their obligations to themselves, to others, and/or to God. Therapists may feel torn between responsibilities to themselves and to patients (e.g., in negotiating boundaries or fees) and between their personal and professional attitudes (e.g., toward homosexuality, abortion, assisted suicide). Third parties such as insurance companies, involved parents, or employers often introduce competing agendas into the treatment. Understanding the process of moral reasoning can help clinicians clarify both the issues at stake and obstacles to resolving them.

Unfair suffering is a common and difficult issue with an important moral dimension. Chapter 5 considers the ways that patients deal with unfair pain through questioning, resignation, blaming themselves, assuming the role of victim, retaliating, seeking public justice, contributing to prevention, or forgiving. To help patients weigh these options, therapists must understand the implications of their own and their patients' world views. They must also remain alert to the ethical and countertransference pitfalls of influencing patients in favor of one option over another.

Chapter 6 considers ways that patients deal with shame and guilt though questioning, rationalization, blame, forgiving themselves, or seeking external forgiveness. How are they to know whether their sense of having failed morally is realistic? When and how should therapists help them make things right? What other resources should they consider enlisting, and how?

Chapter 7 explores the clinical significance of moral growth and transformation. Many individuals facing death, recovering from addiction, and searching for existential or spiritual direction experience profound changes for the better. Demoralized individuals may also look to a therapist for help in reformulating their ideals. What is the role of a clinician in this process? What challenges to ethics and boundaries does encouraging moral change present?

Finally, Chapter 8 considers the relevance of a moral paradigm for helping patients and clinicians achieve authenticity. Not only does each healing paradigm (biological, developmental, intrapsychic, relational, etc.) have important moral aspects, but clinicians are often split (both within and among themselves) in the ways they deliver care, think about the mind versus body and the boundaries of the clinical enterprise, and live out their personal versus professional lives. There are a number of ways that a moral perspective can help clinicians address not only these larger issues but also the practical challenges of learning and teaching about the human condition in full.

Many, but not all, of the illustrative case examples come from my own practice, with nonessential details altered to protect the identities of individuals involved. In some examples, the moral issue is not the central focus of the treatment, and the case can be understood or conceptualized using a "nonmoral" framework as well. Pronouns such as *he* and *she* are used interchangeably rather than the more cumbersome *she/he* throughout.

References

Alonso A: Toward a new understanding of neutrality, in Understanding Therapeutic Action: Psychodynamic Concepts of Cure. Edited by Lifson LE. Hillsdale, NJ, Analytic Press, 1996, pp 3–20

Cushman P: Constructing the Self, Constructing America: A Cultural History of Psychotherapy. New York, Addison-Wesley, 1995

Doherty WJ: Soul Searching: Why Psychotherapy Must Promote Moral Responsibility. New York, Basic Books, 1995

Gedo J: Conceptual Issues in Psychoanalysis. Hillsdale, NJ, Analytic Press, 1986

Gilligan J: Beyond morality: psychoanalytic reflections on shame, guilt and love, in Moral Development and Behavior: Theory, Research and Social Issues. Edited by Likona T, Geis G, Kohlberg L. New York, Holt, Rinehart & Winston, 1976, pp 144–158

Hoffer A: The Freud-Ferenczi controversy—a living legacy. International Review of Psychoanalysis 18:465–472, 1991

Jensen JP, Bergin AE: Mental health values of professional therapists: a national interdisciplinary survey. Professional Psychology Research and Practice 19:290–297, 1988

Lomas P: Doing Good? Psychotherapy Out of Its Depth. New York, Oxford University Press, 1999

Nicholas MW: The Mystery of Goodness and the Positive Moral Consequences of Psychotherapy. New York, WW Norton, 1994

Pellegrino ED, Thomasma DC: The Virtues in Medical Practice. Oxford, England, Oxford University Press, 1993

Pellegrino ED, Thomasma DC: Helping and Healing: Religious Commitment in Health Care. Washington, DC, Georgetown University Press, 1997, pp 97–98

Stone AA: Law, Psychiatry, and Morality: Essays and Analysis. Washington, DC, American Psychiatric Press, 1984

Will OA: Values and the psychotherapist. Am J Psychoanal 41:203–212, 1981

Acknowledgments

U nforgettable discussions with residents in the Harvard Psychiatry Residency Training Program inspired this book. Several colleagues encouraged it in embryonic form, particularly Russ Phillips, Kristine Lima, Allan Josephson, Mary McCarthy, Steve Evans, and Jonathan Borus. Scott Kim nurtured it, reminding me throughout to be clear.

My original editor, Carol Nadelson, accepted and helped the project take shape, and her successor, Bob Hales, skillfully saw it through.

Kristin Lang, Martha Jurchak, Kay Barned Smith, David Hwang, and Paul Guttry each carefully read the manuscript and contributed immeasurably to its final form.

My wife Jean and our three children generously gave me time to write.

CHAPTER

1

Beyond Neutrality

Moral Functioning as a Basis for Therapeutic Influence

> Moral neutrality is not the same as technical neutrality.
>
> Judith Herman, M.D.

Friends give advice, but therapists help patients make their own decisions. This traditional conception of therapeutic neutrality is compelling because clinicians feel responsible for the protection and enhancement of their patients' autonomy. Yet clinicians also need to influence patients. Not only do they intervene to protect patients in acute danger (civil commitment is the most accepted case), but they also inevitably and often appropriately advocate health-related values such as responsibility and relatedness to others (Bergin 1991; Kelly and Strupp 1992; Stone 1984; Tjeltveit 1986). (Various psychotherapeutic schools espouse differing health-related values that express their particular visions of optimal human functioning; see Lakin 1988; London 1986.)

One way of dealing with the fundamental ethical tension between neutrality and influence has been simply to eschew influence. Nondirective schools such as orthodox psychoanalysis and Rogers' client-centered therapy are those best known for cautioning therapists to minimize their impact on patients' values by keeping their own commitments out of sight. However, without accepted ways of owning their positive impact on patients, these therapies have remained specialized forms of intervention rather than ways of providing comprehensive clinical care.

Another approach to resolving this tension has been to attempt informed consent for psychotherapy—that is, obtaining patients' agreement to accept the risk of influence as they would the risks of any other medical procedure. However, even those who emphasize this approach concede that knowing when and how to disclose a therapist's values is, practically speaking, very complicated (Beahrs et al. 2001; Sider 1984; Tjeltveit 1986, 1999; Veatch 1995).

A third approach has been to downplay autonomy as an ideal by suggesting that it may not be either desirable or realistic for patients to make treatment decisions. There is considerable evidence to suggest that patients and families want from their clinicians kindness and competence more than full responsibility for making medical decisions (Schneider 1998). A psychotherapist's influence is not only inevitable and pervasive but also frequently necessary to achieve therapeutic change (Kultgen 1995). Many severely ill patients rely on a therapist's attitudes and actions to structure the treatment relationship. Their therapists' concern, demonstrated by intervening to offer protection, may be crucially important and matter even more than words (Gutheil 1982). Even for healthier patients, a therapist's voice may continue to reverberate even after treatment has ended, raising questions, suggesting alternative perspectives, or offering direction. Although it is a useful corrective to value neutrality, this approach leaves unanswered the question of when it is appropriate and when it is paternalistic for a therapist to exert her moral influence. It also leaves unexamined the value assumptions of the therapist that influence her direction.

A fourth approach is to distinguish between technical and moral neutrality (Caplan 1993; Herman 1992). In other words, a therapist might adopt an even-handed approach to a particular issue without trying to pretend that he is indifferent to which choice the patient makes. Rather than adopting such a position out of loyalty to an ideal of equipoise or one of maximizing the patient's independence, he might have one or more pragmatic, technical reasons for doing so. He might see a need for the patient to improve her decision-making ability. He might recognize that the patient will need to live with the consequences of her decisions. He might act out of respect for the limitations of his own ability to know what is best for her (Hoffer 1985), or he might recognize that they lack informed consent to focus on a controversial issue, given that his and the patient's values differ in important ways. For example, in working with an active alcoholic, a therapist might make clear the advantages of sobriety and urge the patient to consider admission to a detoxification unit while also exploring her ambivalence and helping her to see that the decision to stop drinking is her own to make (Shaffer 1994). This model better defines a time and place for tactical neutrality but does not offer a framework for helping the morally committed therapist act at other times.

Each of these approaches to the problem of moral influence is potentially helpful but fails to provide such a framework. The question remains: If as a general rule it is impossible to be morally neutral in providing therapy but it is unethical to be covertly directive, can clinicians agree on a comprehensive psychotherapeutic ideal that will inform their efforts to help patients live better—more effective, healthier, and happier—lives?

Most clinicians would agree that they should relieve symptoms, restore healthy functioning, and (at least in some cases) promote growth. Most would also agree that they should help patients to make decisions, find their direction, and live in the best possible way. These goals concern what is good and best. As moral ends, they raise the question of how individuals function to achieve them. The rest of this chapter considers how the capacities essential for moral functioning develop and what symptoms result from problems in the way that individuals function morally.

Central to moral functioning is the concept of conscience, or, for dynamically oriented clinicians, the superego. Originally derived from Latin, the term *conscience* implies an inner observing as well as an acting self (Lewis 1960) and performs three overlapping functions: 1) prohibiting wrong behavior through the induction of negative moral emotions such as guilt; 2) promoting positive behavior through the influence of moral commitments embodied in the ego ideal; and 3) applying moral judgment, or the capacity for discriminating and prioritizing competing values.

Freud's concept of the superego as the internalized legacy of early object relationships is very useful clinically in tracing interpersonal influences on the way that patients experience guilt, shame, and obligation. However, as a basis for thinking broadly about what it takes to live morally, it has two major limitations. First, the traditional concept of the superego does not easily accommodate what researchers in other disciplines have learned about the importance of positive emotions (e.g., empathy and concern), shared beliefs (e.g., religious worldviews), and social factors (e.g., cultural biases) in moral functioning. This may be due to the fact that the superego was originally defined as a child's response to the threat of being unloved rather than as her growing appreciation for what is worth loving. Without direct reference to the concept of the superego and using nonclinical populations, developmental psychologists have recently formulated a relatively comprehensive model of moral development that integrates personality, affective, and cognitive variables (Damon 1988; Kohlberg 1983; Rest 1984; Stilwell et al. 1991). Social psychologists have pointed out the ways that historical and cultural factors influence moral attitudes (Kurtines and Gewirtz 1984; Wuthnow 1994). A number of biologists (Alexander 1987; Dawkins 1989; Dennett 1995; Wright 1994), anthropologists (Brown 1991), linguists (Lakoff 1996; Lakoff and Johnson 1980), and philosophers (Hundert 1995; Johnson 1993; Kass 1994; Kovesi 1967; Taylor 1989; Tierney 1994; Wilson 1993) have added further to our understanding of the nature and place of morality in human life.

A second limitation is that the functions traditionally attributed to the superego are primarily evaluative rather than comprehensive. They account less well for how people accomplish other important moral tasks, such as living in accord with their convictions and dealing effectively with their failures to do so. Put in psychoanalytic terms, "it is ego strength rather than superego that results in moral behavior" (Pattison 1969, p. 102).

What, then, are the basic abilities needed to live morally—that is, to achieve moral ends? A person must 1) develop core moral commitments, 2) make decisions based on these commitments, 3) implement these moral decisions, 4) assess the correspondence between behavior and ideals, 5) deal effectively with moral failure, and 6) acquire morally admirable or virtuous character traits. As a suggested framework for understanding the clinician's role, consider next how each of these capacities develops, what factors distort its normal development, and how problems in accomplishing each task can present clinically.

Developing Moral Commitments

Moral commitments refer to a person's core values, such as fairness, freedom, honesty, or concern for others. They define the kind of person one hopes to become and what he believes he ought to do. As such, they are basic to self-regard, identity, and self-esteem (Wuthnow 1994).

In one sense, we choose (consciously or not) our moral commitments, but in the sense that we believe they are universal, they also lay claims of obligation on us. For instance, if I am morally committed to truth telling, I will believe it is also right for others to be truthful and that it is better in some real, objective sense to tell the truth (Taylor 1989). In this way, moral commitments differ from valued preferences: I may avoid eating meat because I prefer to be healthy, whereas if I believe it is wrong to kill animals for food, I will regard this as a principle that others should observe (Rozin 1997). In this way, moral commitments lay claim on other individuals, too, because such commitments are tied to a larger orienting social and philosophical frame of reference.

Moral commitments have both a cognitive and an affective dimension. They are cognitive in that they are concerned with the principles that underlie one's personal goals and beliefs (Kreitler and Kreitler 1976; Raynor and McFarlin 1986). Because these principles provide orientation and direction, they constitute a basis for self-evaluation and corrective changes in course. On the other hand, they also inform and are shaped by what are sometimes known as "moral" emotions, such as compassion, humiliation, and disgust (Margalit 2002; Nussbaum 2001; Rozin 1997).

How do moral commitments develop? It seems likely that a child's sense of what is good originates in preconceptual experiences of empathy, shame, disgust, and guilt (Coles 1997; Damon 1984, 1988; Kurtines and Gewirtz 1984; Nucci 1989) made possible by the limbic system of the mammalian brain (Lewis et al. 2000). These early experiences are themselves influenced both by temperament and the care-taking environment; for example, a basic sense of goodness and badness (both of the self and of others) probably has origins in one's experience with the mother as gratifying or frustrating.[1]

Research on nonclinical populations of children suggests a progression in the way they experience what is good and right. Building on the earlier work of Kohlberg et al., Stilwell et al. (1991) have identified five stages of the process by which children think about morality between ages 5 and 17 years. These stages differ cognitively and anchor the affective, relational, and volitional components of the way children develop their moral commitments.

---

[1]Object relations theorists suggest that split-apart "good" or "bad" internal representations of the self and others normally come together over time, contributing to one's capacity to love and respect others as separate, differentiated individuals and to regard oneself in similar ways (Klein 1948; Schafer 1992; Segal 1974).

In the *External* stage, moral mandates are prelogical and learned through behavioral consequences. A child's sense of what is right and fair is shaped by the process of sharing with others, often sharpened by the experience of unfairness. Permissive or authoritarian parental styles, various cultural emphases, and differing family rules or religious identifications can all exert powerful and nuanced effects during this period (Coles 1986; Kohlberg 1983). By age 7 years, most children have begun to take pride in recounting stored moral rules and experience a sense of personal goodness by following them (the *Heart/Brain* stage). Older children, ages 11–13 years, begin to integrate moral feelings and rules by personifying the conscience as a resource for consulting in making decisions (the *Heart/ Mind* stage). Midadolescents struggle to resolve conflicting mandates coming from peers, authorities, and popular culture (the *Confused* stage, corresponding to Freud's phase of oedipal conflict). Older adolescents at the *Integrated* stage experience a degree of comfort with some ambiguity in moral rules and a greater necessity for personal decision making.

As an adolescent's moral commitments are consolidated, refined, and nurtured over the course of adulthood through the influence of mentors and heroes and her community and spiritual life (Colby and Damon 1992), they form the basis of her ideal moral self or ego ideal (Chassequet-Smirgel 1976; McGlashan and Miller 1982; Milrod 1990). Normally, moral commitments are sufficiently integrated with a mature individual's view of reality that they allow her to master difficult moral dilemmas or withstand a challenge to her identity, such as that presented by a serious illness (Viederman and Perry 1980).

Obviously many factors can interfere with the development of moral commitments. As Stilwell et al. (1994) point out, moral responsiveness requires an awareness of the emotional arousal associated with events that evoke a sense of "oughtness" (whether positively resulting in pride or elation or negatively resulting in the experience of guilt or shame). Hence excesses or deficiencies of anxiety and problems in mood regulation may correlate with moral delay, arrest, or deviancy (Stilwell et al. 1994). For example, constitutional difficulties in handling anxiety (Kagan et al. 1988a, 1988b) may predispose a child to react to developmental challenges conservatively or defensively, with a corresponding effect on his moral commitments. More specifically, children with excessive anxiety from infancy might be expected to show good inhibitory moral capacity but difficulty developing the courage and peace that mastery of anxiety fosters in later development. By contrast, children who appear deficient in anxiety show less fear of punishment, may have difficulty responding to censure, and may be more likely to develop in an antisocial direction (Quay et al. 1987).

Because the development of moral commitments depends on internalization, empathy, sympathy, and examples of fairness, relationships are crucial. Neglect in early childhood can inhibit the normal unfolding of the child's capacity for empathy. Early sexual abuse may confuse the victim about what is right. Unfair treatment can contribute to cynicism or to a search for vindication. Arbitrary, harsh, or inconsistent parenting may engender rebellion against authority, inability to identify with societal values, and delinquency (Glueck and Glueck 1950; Samson and Laub 1993). On the other hand, overly permissive parenting may contribute to lax expectations and inconsistent standards that are characteristic of "superego lacunae" (Johnson and Szurek 1952). Religious training that is harsh or inconsistent may retard identification with positive ideals; negative role models and peer group experiences (especially during adolescence) can encourage antisocial attitudes.

Cultures and subcultures can mediate values that if unexamined make racism, sexism, or violence ego-syntonic (Hamilton 1971; Margalit 2002; Rabkin 1975). An example familiar to many clinicians is the ideal of dutiful self-denial for women upheld by many paradigms of traditional marriage (Costello 1977; Gilligan 1993).

Finally, unexamined and/or unresolved conflict between cultural, religious, parental, or other values may interfere with the appropriation and integration of a person's ideals. Consider the wide range of moral attitudes held by Americans: Individualistic utilitarianism stresses the importance of practical consequences to the individual; corporate utilitarianism gives priority to the organization to which one is loyal; emotivism emphasizes feelings as the standard for determining what is right and good; altruism takes the well-being of others as an important consideration; moral absolutism emphasizes the importance of underlying principles or standards; and theistic moralism both grounds moral standards in a view of God and asserts the importance of serving God (Wuthnow 1994). When individuals do think more deeply about how to ground their own commitments, they are often torn between appeals from on the one hand those who emphasize autonomy and personal choice in identifying values and on the other those who see moral principles as rooted more fundamentally—for example, in a spiritual worldview (Kurtines and Gewirtz 1984).

What is the clinical importance of moral commitments? Uncertainty regarding core values can contribute to disturbances in identity and fluctuations in self-esteem in situations such as adolescent turmoil (Schonfeld 1971), adjustment to medical illness (Viederman and Perry 1980), and recovery from trauma (Herman 1992) and addiction (Akhtar 1984). Clinicians treating patients with these conditions often must help them review, reconceptualize, or consolidate their moral commitments (Cooper 1972; May 1975; Pattison 1969). They may also help their patients find constructive uses for their newly consolidated commitments to fairness or to preventing others from experiencing what they have suffered.

> A second-year medical student came for treatment because of difficulty concentrating on her work and doubts about staying in medicine. As the oldest child of a physician in an Asian family, she had always felt considerable pressure (which she described as cultural) to do well in school and follow parental direction. These values received additional moral weight from the conservative church to which the family belonged. They went unquestioned until she learned that her father had concealed for several months her mother's recurrence of cancer to avoid interfering with her completion of the medical school term. At that point she became acutely disillusioned with her parents' commitment to education but experienced difficulty articulating her own. She took a leave of absence and sought treatment to help clarify what she cared most about before deciding whether to return to school.

Clinicians working with patients at points of important transition, such as the end of life, have begun to recognize the importance of their moral commitments. For example, E. H. Cassem (personal communication, November 1999) has suggested questions such as the following for eliciting what matters most to a patient:

- How would you describe yourself?
- What sort of person are you?
- How do/would you like to be thought of?
- Is there anyone whose needs you would put ahead of your own?
- What are your goals/dreams in life?
- Looking back, is there anything you are especially proud of?
- Do you have a philosophy of life or a code that you live by?
- If virtues are important to you, how would you rank loyalty, honesty, compassion, love, courage, and so forth?
- What would you say that you stand for?
- Is there anything in your life worth dying for?
- What is the time when you have laughed the hardest?

Such questions help clarify the values patients will need to call upon in making difficult decisions.

Making Moral Decisions

There are several steps in the process of reasoning morally or using one's commitments to make decisions (Rest 1986). The first step is interpreting the situation, including ascertaining the facts of the case and recognizing the presence of a moral problem. This recognition depends in turn on the ability to imagine oneself in the roles of the different participants in the situation and to assess how each is affected by various actions. For example, antisocial individuals often lack empathy, preventing them from appreciating the needs of others.

A second step is envisioning possible approaches to solving the moral problem. Kohlberg (1983) and his colleagues are best known for having extended Piaget's (1932) observation that children progressively develop in their ability to conceive solutions to moral problems. The sequential reasoning patterns that Kohlberg identified have since become known as punishment and obedience (social Darwinism), instrumentalism (Machiavellianism), popular conformity, allegiance to authority, social contract (democratic participation), and universality of ethical principles. Kohlberg and Ryncarz (1990) have proposed a seventh, "softer" stage, during which an individual relates morality to an ontological or cosmic orientation that answers the question "Why be moral?" Stilwell et al. (1994) have documented a similar progressive unfolding in the capacity of children for moral conceptualization.

Gender and culture can influence the alternatives that individuals envision. For example, Gilligan (1993) has shown that men more frequently focus on considerations of justice, whereas women tend to be more concerned with considerations of care for others. Political conservatives and liberals often reason morally in different ways, which Lakoff (1996) has compared to authoritarian and permissive parental styles.

Patients struggling with a life decision often have difficulty envisioning possible approaches that are consistent with their values.

A 30-year-old secretary became strongly attracted to her boss as he was leaving the company. They had an affair, and she moved in with him. Shortly afterward, she consulted a psychiatrist, indecisive about whether she should divorce her husband, to whom she felt loyal but whom she described as "boring." At her initial appointment, she revealed that her desire to embark on a new life with her ex-boss was primarily hampered by her belief that divorce was wrong. When asked about this, she responded that her belief came from the teaching of the nuns in her parochial school.

Exploration revealed that she was struggling with both conflicting feelings about her husband and ambivalence toward the religious authority that the nuns represented. Specifically, she could neither reject their teachings outright nor identify enough with their belief system to formulate her own differentiated understanding of marriage and divorce within a religious worldview.

In addition to exploring this patient's feelings, her therapist helped her see that because her moral reasoning was arrested at the stage of allegiance to authority, she was having difficulty envisioning possible justifications for alternative plans of action.

A third, relatively complex step in moral reasoning is deciding which of several possible courses of action best fit one's ideals and what to actually do. It involves knowing one's moral commitments (e.g., to self-interest, personal values, religious obligations, universal rules, utilitarian benefits) and applying them through the use of imagination, checklists, questions, or some less formal methodology (Worthey 1997). The more conscious or intentional this process, the less likely that one will do, for example, an unselfish thing for masochistic reasons or, conversely, a harmful thing from good but misguided intentions. It also involves emotional engagement (Greene et al. 2001; Nussbaum 2001). Individuals with difficulty attending or taking initiative can falter at this point.

An Italian-American laborer referred for depression after a serious heart attack felt torn for years between loyalty to his aged mother with whom he lived and his obligation to his 10-year-old daughter, who was living with his estranged wife in Italy. He was preoccupied with whether he should now move overseas and leave his mother, visit his daughter more often, or insist that his mother move with him to Italy. While he could identify his overriding commitments (the interests of both of his loved ones) and anticipate the probable consequences of the alternatives (e.g., how each person would feel in the short and long term), he seemed hopeless that anything in his life could work out. His psychiatrist acknowledged that he faced a serious moral problem and helped him to see that much of his indecisiveness was due to his depression. When he felt better physically and more himself emotionally, he could begin to explore a move to Italy.

Implementing Moral Decisions

Unless acted on, moral decisions have little value. We associate implementation with the capacities to defer gratification, control competing impulses, anticipate vulnerability, and enlist help when needed. Yet people with considerable ego strength fail to do what they know they should. Consider the example of U.S. President Clinton's behavior with White House intern Monica Lewinsky.

The problem of evil or moral failure has fascinated thinkers from a variety of disciplines throughout history (Levine 1997). The theological doctrine of the Devil and Freud's theory of the death instinct emphasize the irrational power of evil. Other explanations stress the importance of weakness or perversity of the will (Kierkegaard 1847/1938). Still others suggest that moral failure begins with succumbing to temptation and continues as a dynamic process involving both instinct and ego, or will (Plantinga 1995). The Achilles' heels of both Shakespeare's Macbeth and Hawthorne's Rev. Dimsdale first made them vulnerable to acting contrary to their convictions. They began to rationalize and/or deny their wrongdoing, then became progressively entangled in a web of deception and corruption. Augustine described his slide from insecurity through grasping, greed, prejudice, intolerance, eventually to cruelty in almost addictive terms: "For out of the perverse will came lust, and the service of lust became habit, and habit, not resisted, became necessity." (Augustine 1955). There is, of course, a social component to both institutionalized evil and to individual patterns of moral failure such as prejudice, intolerance, and the other forms of entitlement that perpetuate abuse (Adorno 1950; Allport 1954; Arendt 1951; Grand 2000; Lamb 1996; Langmuir 1990; Young-Bruehl 1996).

After lagging behind disciplines such as philosophy, theology, literature, and sociology, the mental health profession has recently devoted increasing scrutiny to relatively severe forms of moral failure such as delinquency, psychopathy (Meloy 1992; Welner 1998), sadism, and "wickedness" (Levine 1997), as well as to conditions such as domestic violence and the failure of clinicians to maintain professional boundaries (Olarte 1991).

> A 55-year-old businessman reluctantly agreed to treatment at the urging of his wife, who had threatened to leave him after 30 years of marriage. He prided himself on being a good provider and caring father but admitted to outbursts during which he had been loud and insulting and had frightened his wife by driving recklessly or threatening suicide. While he typically apologized and behaved considerately for some weeks after each incident, she had decided she was no longer willing to live in fear.

Under his wife's pressure, this patient acknowledged that his behavior was wrong but at first rationalized that it was provoked. His therapist's support for facing the wrongfulness of his behavior opened the door for him to take more responsibility and to look at what made him vulnerable to losing control. He realized that he felt angry and helpless whenever he sensed that his wife was adopting a superior attitude, reminiscent of the critical condemnation he felt from his mother that had left him feeling insecure and frustrated as a child.

From working with destructive people, Goldberg (2000) has developed one of the most comprehensive formulations of the factors involved in the development of delinquency and violence. These include vulnerability to shame, benign parental neglect, inability to mourn, linguistic difficulties expressing feelings, and witnessing significant people who behave as if rageful anger were a legitimate means for dealing with frustration and conflict.

Assessing One's Behavior

Different ego states indicate to a person whether he or she is doing the right thing. Normally, pride reflects a positive self-assessment in relation to one's ideal self, and self-esteem depends on maintaining this positive correspondence between one's perceived self and ego ideal (Kernberg 1976). Conversely, a sense of guilt, shame, or remorse over sin signals moral failure (Higgins et al. 1985). Individuals feel *guilt* when they transgress commitments that they have internalized as standards (or in psychoanalytic terms, as injunctions of the superego). *Shame* and loss of self-esteem result when people fail to live up to their ideals or to positive obligations to do or be good (Morrison 1989; Piers and Singer 1971), especially in relation to a real or imagined audience (Bupp 1983; Singer, in Piers and Singer 1971). Like remorse, they are indications that a person takes his commitments seriously (Greenspan 1995). The concepts of shame and guilt sometimes overlap (Kugler and Jones 1992). For example, Heidegger, Kierkegaard, Tillich, May, and Yalom refer to existential guilt, or a sense of "anxious badness" that results from a sense of transgression against the self because of having failed to fulfill possibility or potentiality.

Sin can imply intentionality or a fractured self but most often implies an offense against a relationship, as suggested by the lines that the Prodigal Son had prepared for his father: "I have sinned against you and against God and am no more worthy to be called your son."

How does the capacity to assess oneself develop? Melanie Klein (1948) and her followers postulated that the infant's experiences of affirmation and rejection by the mother are early precursors of pride or shame and guilt, respectively. The research of Stilwell et al. (1994) suggests that children normally learn to apply moral commitments and reasoning to their own actions and to tolerate the distress of shame or guilt in a stepwise fashion. Before age 7 years, they are concerned mainly with fear of punishment or rejection after wrongdoing defined by adults. Between ages 7 and 11 years, children internalize rules of conscience sufficiently to cause feelings of anxiety in the absence of anyone else knowing about a particular misdeed. Stilwell et al. showed that young teenagers use memories of past misdeeds to conduct a moral review and experience more prolonged periods of distress (e.g., feelings of guilt, loss of energy, or social withdrawal) in relation to moral transgression. They further point out that psychophysiological sensitivity (e.g., loss of appetite, stomachaches, headaches, loss of sleep) to moral issues develops around this time and increases during midadolescence. During later adolescence, individuals begin to feel pride in meeting a moral challenge and use an increasing capacity for introspection to anticipate how a hypothetical moral failure is likely to produce bodily symptoms. In these ways, shame and guilt come to serve important restraining functions (Lamb 1996; Morrison 1989).

Clinicians are familiar with the fact that various clinical conditions can distort self-assessment. Depression is the most common (Prosen et al. 1983): exaggerated guilt and recrimination are among the most painful symptoms of patients who are seriously depressed. Psychodynamic explanations for depressive guilt include Freud's (1917/1957) hypothesis that it represents anger turned inward and Klein's (1948) formulation that the individual in the "depressive position" feels guilt because he recognizes that his destructive impulses could destroy the object on which he depends (Segal 1974). However, the fact that irrational guilt disappears when major depression responds to somatic treatment suggests that biological factors are equally important.

Survivors of trauma, whether from combat or sexual abuse, may also show an exaggerated sense of shame and responsibility and even of unworthiness to receive help (Herman 1992; Kernberg 1976; Lamb 1996; Modell 1965).

A 30-year-old day-care worker who had been sexually abused and physically intimidated by her father for years came for treatment during his terminal illness. Her suicidal ideation, anorexia, purging, alcohol abuse, and self-cutting eventually stabilized, but her feelings of shame and guilt remained. At her work, she overextended herself on behalf of abused children, whom she saw as victims of adult mistreatment and not (as she saw herself) responsible for their plight.

Patients with obsessive-compulsive disorder (OCD) may suffer from overly severe self-assessment in the form of an irrational preoccupation with imaginary sins.

An athletic, well-liked high school senior in a religious family became preoccupied with having had occasional homosexual urges and of being guilty of an unpardonable sin. His concerns were inconsistent with both the teachings of his church and his own premorbid beliefs and responded well to a trial of clomipramine.

Rapoport et al. (1989) proposed links between such patients' guilt and fear about sexual or religious transgressions and disturbances in those brain circuits connecting the basal ganglia with the frontal lobes, which are concerned with rule-governed behavior. They cited for support both the presence of serotonin in these pathways and the effectiveness of serotonergic agents in treating OCD. Distinguishing the scrupulosity of obsessional patients who "repent when they have not sinned" from religious guilt or shame can be a diagnostic challenge (Suess and Halpern 1989).

In contrast, impairment of frontal and limbic functioning found in states such as mania and intoxication are often associated with overly lax self-assessment ("the superego is soluble in alcohol"). Batterers (who have often been abused themselves), individuals with superego lacunae (Aldrich 1987; Johnson and Szurek 1952; Singer 1974), and those with psychopathic traits may not feel appropriate guilt, instead rationalizing their various forms of exploitation, cheating, and sexual harassment.

Dealing With Moral Failure

Addressing moral failure enables people to both satisfy their sense of justice and remain identified with what is good (Dyer 1988; Finkelstein 1991).

Stilwell et al. (1994) documented how children heal after a painful moral failure. Under age 7 years, they typically make a quick admission of wrongdoing, wish they could undo it, and quickly forget. Between ages 7 and 11 years, they are likely to find comfort in disciplinary action, attempts at speedy reparation and reconciliation, and promises of reform. At this stage they may ascribe healing to these actions or to other factors such as sleep, time, or food. The behavior of young teenagers is more complex. They may seek advice from respected adults and appreciate the benefits of listening to music, reading, or showing affection toward an offended person. Midadolescents may persist in communicating with an offended party despite feeling embarrassed or ashamed, compensate with alternative good deeds, or participate in religious rituals of reconciliation. Older adolescents tend to engage in "soul searching" as well as activities such as exercise, room cleaning, journal writing, or drawing. Young adults, able to appreciate that full reparation may never be possible, begin to find ways of living with past mistakes. They may engage in constructive activities such as strengthening attachment to family and friends, appreciate the value of reestablishing trust after a breach, and develop self-deprecating humor. As adults they may also deal with guilt through socially imposed penalties (such as restitution, a fine, or a prison sentence) and self-imposed ones (such as sacrifice, penance, or apology).

Dealing effectively with shame may require one to change direction. For example, religious conversion provides a way to go from a searching reevaluation of the self to identification with a new moral vision (James 1903/1958). Moving encounters with human grace can also catalyze repentance and moral reorientation, as in Jean Valjean's experience with the bishop in Victor Hugo's *Les Miserables*.

Repairing a relationship damaged by wrongdoing may require forgiveness. Once considered the province of theologians, forgiveness of oneself and others has recently attracted serious attention from both social scientists and clinicians (Gartner 1988; Hargrave 1994; Hope 1987; McCullough et al. 2000; Richards and Bergin 1997; Smedes 1984; Worthington 1998).

The process of forgiveness begins with the recognition that one has suffered unfairly. Honesty about being hurt is a necessary first step toward possible reconciliation (as seen in South Africa's Truth and Reconciliation Commission, chaired by Archbishop Desmond Tutu). Later, a survivor's memory of pain may enable her to empathize with potential victims and engage in social activism (Higgins 1994; Margalit 2002).

Genuine forgiveness also involves feeling anger, or a wish that the offender suffer. An incest survivor may want to forget, but as Rose in Jane Smiley's novel *A Thousand Acres* notes, forgiveness is more than "a reflex for when you can't stand what you know."

A third crucial step in the process of forgiveness is mastering emotions such as resentment and humiliation (Margalit 2002; Schimmel 2002) in order to develop a different attitude toward an offender as someone who is, for example, limited, needy, and human, though still morally accountable. An apology can facilitate this shift in attitude but is not always necessary. For many individuals, a larger context of meaning helps them to view both themselves and others as in need of forgiveness (Jones 1995).[2]

Finally, a readiness for reconciliation depends on restitution and/or changed behavior. Polarized spouses are likely to require concrete evidence of change before they can begin to trust again. In political life, adversaries negotiate verifiable conditions for peace. In religious life,

---

[2]De Waal (1996) described a precursor of this phase in those higher primates who, apparently mindful of the partner's value, engage in a process of respectful negotiation of the relationship that he called "strategic reconciliation."

reconciliation with God or another supreme being may require sacrifice and/or the initiation of a new way of life; examples include participation in the Jewish Day of Atonement, Christian confession, and Muslim prayer or observance of Ramadan.

Problems in dealing with moral failure can present as intractable guilt or shame, moralism, bitterness ("fondled hatreds," in C.S. Lewis's words), estrangement, and denial, which Kierkegaard (1849/1968) called the "sickness unto death" (Mullen 1981). Anna Freud's remarks about a case presented to her by Robert Coles (1988, p. 180), in which the patient was a widow who remained angry, difficult, and embittered after years of therapy, indicate how difficult it can be to help these patients within the context of traditional psychotherapy:

> I will confess to you: when I was listening to all of this, I thought to myself that this poor old lady doesn't need us at all. No, she's had her fill of "us," even if she doesn't know it. She's been visiting one or another of "us" for years, decades, as she has dealt with her son's troubles, her husband's, her own. What she needs, I thought, is forgiveness. She needs to make peace with her soul, not talk about her mind. There must be a God, somewhere, to help her, to hear her, to heal her—so I thought for a second! But I fear she'll not find him!

Chapters 5 and 6 consider ways that clinicians can help patients to deal with their own and others' moral failure.

Developing Virtues

All cultures share a remarkably consistent vision of optimal human behavior (Lewis 1947). For example, five traits of a good person are so basic that they have traditionally become known as the cardinal virtues: 1) fairness, 2) courage, 3) conscientiousness or integrity (which Rawls [1971] described as "truthfulness and sincerity, humility and commitment, or . . . authenticity"), 4) prudence (or practical wisdom), and 5) self-control. Other traits important to living well include generosity, mercy, compassion, humility, simplicity, tolerance, purity, and gentleness (Comte-Sponville 2001).

During the early part of the twentieth century, in part because the Victorians associated the virtues with respectability, the concept of virtue was eclipsed by more neutral concepts such as values and moral reasoning (Himmelfarb 1995). However, since the 1980s, there has been a broad resurgence of interest in the virtues. Psychologists have begun to integrate virtue-based models with stage-based models of moral maturity (Power et al. 1989). Educators have called for character education, understood as the training of students in the character traits that are essential to a good life in a good society (Ryan and McLean 1987). Contemporary philosophers (MacIntyre 1984; Slote 1992) and ethicists (Beauchamp and Childress 2001) have emphasized the importance of virtuous character in producing moral behavior. A subcommittee of the American Board of Internal Medicine recommended in 1983 that residency directors rigorously evaluate physicians for the essential humanistic qualities of integrity, respect, and compassion. Additionally, a growing number of mental health professionals have identified the enhancement of virtues as one of the goals of psychotherapy (Doherty 1995; Lagerman 1993; Nicholas 1994; Weiner 1993).

Mental health professionals have been somewhat reluctant to discuss virtues in relation to clinical work for four possible reasons. First, lists of virtues can sound like dry, abstract principles that have only a tangential relationship to the concerns of patients. Yet as core aspects of their identity, virtues express both patients' beliefs about reality (Parekh 1993, p. 60; Porter 1995; Streng 1993) and their beliefs about the kind of people they want to become (Colby and Damon 1992; Stilwell et al. 1998). Someone who characteristically acts out of concern for others is usually not simply following a principle but a deeply felt commitment. Pellegrino and Thomasma (1996) described what this means for a physician with a Christian understanding of the medical virtues:

> Autonomy becomes more than a negative prerogative; it becomes a positive respect for the enormous dignity of the patient as a child of God who has autonomy because of God-given dignity. Humans have dignity not because they are autonomous but because they are humans. Justice becomes charitable justice not by the strict weighing of what is owed by rule of law but by the rule of charity. (p. 25)

A second reason for clinicians' reluctance to use the language of virtue is the relationship between virtues and particular systems of belief. Individuals whom we consider virtuous tend to show an unusual degree of integration not only between their behavior and their ideals but among personal, social, and spiritual factors. For example, Colby and Damon (1992) found, in studying moral exemplars, that these factors included hopefulness, positivity (linked with the ability to forgive the self and others), a dynamic relationship with a community of support, and a transcendent belief (for many, though not all, this belief rested in God as a force for good). Yet patients' worldviews and spiritual lives are often neglected in clinical exploration, and clinicians are frequently uncertain how to relate their own worldview to their work (Schultz-Ross and Gutheil 1997).

A third reason may be that virtues are often seen as only "other-regarding," or "prosocial" traits, so that advocating them can feel moralistic. In fact, many virtues are "self-regarding" (e.g., self-respect or prudence), and all virtues inform and express attitudes toward the self as well as toward others (Parekh 1993; Porter 1995; Slote 1992). Altruism is a "mature" character trait because it is good for oneself as well as for others (Dyer 1986; Vaillant 1977).

Yet a fourth reason that therapists tend not to incorporate concepts of virtue into their clinical approach may be their own lack of reflection about their own moral view (Nicholas 1994). This can contribute to reluctance to address the topic with a patient.

Despite their avoidance of the term *virtue*, mental health professionals have been interested in the development of *character*, which, as Aristotle pointed out, begins with an individual's temperament. The research of Cloninger et al. (1993) has distinguished four dimensions of temperament that are independently heritable, evident early in life, and involve preconceptual biases in perceptual memory and habit formation: novelty seeking, harm avoidance, reward dependence, and persistence. Cloninger has made a plausible case that these form the basis for the maturing of character along three directions: *self-directedness,* the extent to which one self-identifies as an autonomous individual; *cooperativeness,* the extent to which one self-identifies as an integral part of humanity; and *self-transcendence,* the extent to which one self-identifies as an integral part of the universe as a whole. These three closely resemble the basic "moral sentiments" described by Wilson (1993): self-control, sympathy, and fairness/duty. It seems likely that these have biological correlates in frontal brain function and in what Lewis et al. (2000) has referred to as "limbic regulation."

Cloninger has presented evidence that a greater degree of *self-directedness*, which can be seen as a self-regarding virtue, is inversely related to the likelihood of developing a personality disorder. The self-directed individual accepts responsibility for his own choices (instead of blaming other people and circumstances), identifies individually valued goals and purposes (instead of lacking goal direction), develops skills and confidence in solving problems or resourcefulness (instead of remaining apathetic), accepts himself (instead of striving), and shows what Cloninger called "congruent second nature" (instead of personal mistrust of his own habits).

Cooperativeness comprises more other-directed virtuous traits: social acceptance (instead of intolerance), empathy (instead of social disinterest), helpfulness (instead of unhelpfulness), compassion (instead of revengefulness), and "pure-hearted principles" (instead of self-advantage).

Self-transcendence often supports the development of other-directed character traits. Cloninger found three aspects of self-transcendence in a broad spectrum of individuals and cultures (not just in rare mystics). SELF-FORGETFUL (instead of self-conscious) experiences refer to getting lost in the moment, detached from time and place, or experiencing a deep oneness with all that exists. TRANSPERSONAL IDENTIFICATION (instead of self-isolation) refers to feeling very connected to nature or wanting to sacrifice to make the world a better place. SPIRITUAL ACCEPTANCE (instead of rational materialism) refers to feeling a spiritual connection to other people that cannot be explained in words, or feeling guided by a spiritual force greater than any human being.

Many internal and external factors influence the development of character along these lines. As a young child's moral emotions, judgment, cognition, and self-understanding mature, he acquires capacities for love and respect (Coles 1997; Damon 1995; Stilwell et al. 1998). Integration of good and bad internalized representations allows him to maintain love (including for himself) and relationships through conflicts and difficulties and to forgive (Gartner 1988; Klein 1948; Schafer 1992; Segal 1974). Conversations or narratives (Hauerwas 1981) and significant relationships (Jones 1990) significantly shape character. Practices such as personal reflection and training may become important (Porter 1995). Lastly, institutions that support spiritual and social practices can play a formative role (MacIntyre 1984).

Individuals with personality disorders lack one or more adaptive (or, one might say, virtuous) character traits. Antisocial personalities lack prosocial virtues almost by definition (Vaillant 1975). Obsessional personalities overvalue control (Mollinger 1980), narcissistic personalities overvalue admiration (Eisnitz 1974; Lax 1989; Tyson and Tyson 1984), and histrionic personalities overvalue attention (Baumbacher and Amini 1980–81).

Doherty (1995), writing as a family therapist in *Soul Searching: Why Psychotherapy Must Promote Moral Responsibility*, addresses with unusual directness the issues involved in helping patients to develop virtues such as commitment, justice, truthfulness, and what he refers to as community. Arguing that the efforts of the conventionally trained therapist to simply show how virtues are in the patient's self-interest are inadequate, Doherty goes further to remind his patients of the existence of obligations to others to be fair, truthful, or faithful. Overholser (1999) and Goldberg (2000) similarly suggest ways of promoting virtue in psychotherapy by emphasizing the importance of a capacity to learn to speak the language of felt emotion, a concern with fairness and justice for others, assuming responsibility for one's own behavior, moral courage, and a willingness to self-examine. Although Doherty's directive to promote virtue directly may seem foreign to many contemporary clinicians, it can be argued that psychiatry throughout its history has embodied virtuous ideals in four important respects.

First, since the time of Hippocrates, the fundamental mission of psychiatry as a part of medicine has been to care in a compassionate and altruistic way for those made vulnerable by illness. The contemporary "Patient-Physician Covenant" (Crawshaw et al. 1995) makes the moral nature of this mission clear:

> Medicine is, at its center, a moral enterprise grounded in a covenant of trust. This covenant obliges physicians to be competent and to use their competence in the patient's best interests. Physicians, therefore, are both intellectually and morally obligated to act as advocates for the sick wherever their welfare is threatened and for their health at all times.

Psychiatric reformers such as Philippe Pinel and Dorothea Dix and later leaders of the Moral Treatment Period (Sederer 1977) not only cared for individual patients but also advocated for more humane treatment for all. Still later, clinicians, including psychiatrists, psychologists, nurses, and social workers, formulated codes of ethics that emphasized the responsibility of practitioners to use their skills on their patients' behalf. Today, both practitioners and their professional organizations actively struggle for parity and equal access to quality care.

Second, in addition to altruistically promoting humane, effective, and equitable care for the mentally ill, psychiatrists promote health-related values, or virtues (Balint and Sheldon 1996; Brock 1991; Emanuel and Emanuel 1992). Those important to mature coping and mental health include honesty, authenticity, responsibility, and care and respect for others and for oneself (Balint 1964; Comfort 1981; Doherty 1995; Greifinger 1997; Mowrer 1967). Virtues particularly important to achieving the goals of group and family therapy include concern for the good of others and acceptance of their values (Mullan 1991; Nicholas 1994).

Of course, various therapeutic schools have emphasized somewhat different values based on implicit concepts of health and human nature (Bergin 1980, 1991; Cushman 1995; Jones 1994; London 1986; Margolis 1966). Such differences, as well as those that exist among the beliefs of individual clinicians, raise important ethical questions, because even a relatively nondirective, "neutral" stance conveys something of the therapist's own attitude and values. These questions include the following:

- How should a clinician recognize and deal with her inevitable influence on her patients' values? (Bergin 1991; Kelly and Strupp 1992)
- What are the limits of a clinician's legitimate role in a patient's life?
- What constitutes undue influence?
- Should the clinician's role in the patient's life depend on whether she and the patient share the same worldview?

The American Psychiatric Association took a first step toward clarifying the relationship between clinicians' personal and professional values in its 1989 "Guidelines Regarding Possible Conflict Between Psychiatrists' Religious Commitments and Psychiatric Practice."

Similar questions arise from the fact that mental health professionals have come to represent for many in our culture a "secular priesthood" and are consulted in areas of human behavior made controversial by conflicting moral and social values, such as sexual norms and assisted suicide (Bellah et al. 1985; Cushman 1995; Hillman and Ventura 1992; Jones 1994; London 1986; Margolis 1966; Rieff 1966). What are the social and political implications of this influence (Halleck 1971; Miller 1976; Rieff 1959; Stone 1984; Szasz 1983)? How are clinicians to deal with the fact that the goals of treatment themselves are often influenced by cultural factors (Gilligan 1993)? For example, how are clinicians to balance the value that Western psychotherapists frequently place on maximizing individual autonomy (Engelhardt 1973) with a concern for relatedness (Miller 1976)? How can therapists guard against succumbing to cultural insensitivity (Spiegel 1971) or contributing to a patient's self-absorbed preoccupation (Miller 1976)?

A third way in which psychiatry has come to embody virtuous ideals is that clinicians themselves must embody certain virtues, such as humility, caring, honesty, and courage (Doherty 1995; Will 1981). For example, patients need to trust that their therapists' integrity and wisdom will enable them to respect confidentiality and maintain therapeutic boundaries (Dyer 1988; Holmes and Lindley 1989; Lakin 1988; Paredes et al. 1990; Stone 1984). Chapter 3 explores further the importance and the development of caring as a professional virtue.

Fourth, psychiatry is concerned with the patient as a whole person, including his moral struggles. Patients grappling with decisions that have moral implications may need help to clarify and apply their values to such decisions (Buhler 1962; Doherty 1995; Macklin 1973). Patients whose trust in people and in a moral order have been damaged by severe trauma may need their clinicians to adopt a committed moral stance (Herman 1992; Lifton 1976).

Many clinicians who would agree that psychiatry deals with moral

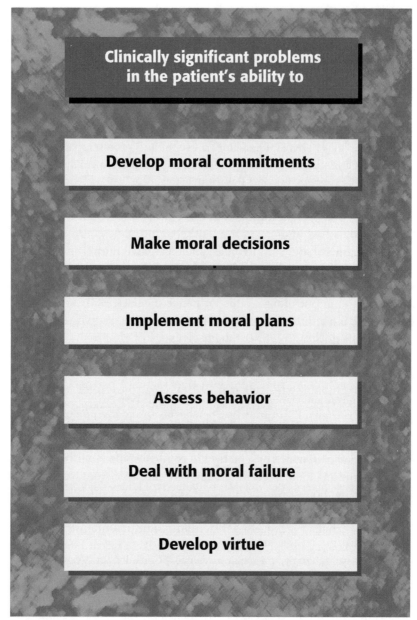

FIGURE 1.   Bases for a clinician's moral influence.

ideals in these four general senses would still question how to integrate the task of acquiring virtues into everyday practice. This chapter offers a paradigm that is based on how people function morally: how they develop moral commitments, make and implement moral decisions, assess and deal with moral failure, and acquire virtues. It has also suggested that identifying problems in a person's moral functioning is the first step toward defining the clinician's role as a moral agent in other aspects of his care (Figure 1). Chapter 2 explores how optimal treatment planning takes the patient's needs and values, as well as the therapist's moral influence, into account.

References

Adorno TW: The Authoritarian Personality. New York, Harper, 1950

Akhtar S: The syndrome of identity diffusion. Am J Psychiatry 141:1381–1385, 1984

Aldrich CK: Acting out and acting up: the superego lacuna revisited. Am J Orthopsychiatry 57:402–406, 1987

Alexander RD: The Biology of Moral Systems. New York, Aldine de Gruyter, 1987

Allport G: The Nature of Prejudice. Cambridge, MA, Addison-Wesley, 1954

Arendt H: The Origins of Totalitarianism. New York, Harcourt Brace, 1951

Augustine: Confessions. Translated and edited by Outler AC. Philadelphia, PA, Westminster, 1955

Balint M: The Doctor, His Patient and the Illness, 2nd Edition. London, Pitman Books, 1964

Balint M: The Basic Fault: Therapeutic Aspects of Regression. London, Tavistock, 1968

Balint M, Shelton W: Regaining the initiative: forging a new model of the patient-physician relationship. JAMA 20:887–891, 1996

Baumbacher G, Amini F: The hysterical personality disorder: a proposed clarification of a diagnostic dilemma. Int J Psychoanal Psychother 8:501–532, 1980–81

Beahrs JO, Gutheil TG: Informed consent in psychotherapy. Am J Psychiatry 158:4–10, 2001

Beauchamp TL, Childress JF: Principles of Biomedical Ethics, 5th Edition. New York, Oxford University Press, 2001

Bellah RN, Madsen R, Sullivan WM, et al: Habits of the Heart: Individualism and Commitment in American Life. Berkeley, University of California Press, 1985

Bergin AE: Psychotherapy and religious values. J Consult Clin Psychol 48:95–105, 1980

Bergin AE: Values and religious issues in psychotherapy and mental health. Am Psychol 46:394–403, 1991

Brock DW: The ideal of shared decision making between physicians and patients. Kennedy Institute of Ethics Journal 1:28–47, 1991

Brown DE: Human Universals. Philadelphia, PA, Temple University Press, 1991

Buhler C: Values in Psychotherapy. Glencoe, IL, Free Press, 1962

Bupp CS: An examination of shame and guilt among veterans of the Vietnam conflict. Unpublished doctoral dissertation, University of Minnesota, Minneapolis, 1983

Caplan AL: Neutrality is not morality: the ethics of genetic counseling, in Prescribing Our Future: Ethical Challenges in Genetic Counseling. Edited by Bartels DM, LeRoy BS, Caplan AL. New York, Aldine de Gruyter, 1993, pp 149–165

Chasseguet-Smirgel J: Some thoughts on the ego ideal: a contribution to the study of the "illness of ideality." Psychoanal Q 45:345–373, 1976

Cloninger CR, Svrakic DM, Prybeck TR: A psychobiological model of temperament and character. Arch Gen Psychiatry 50:975–990, 1993

Colby A, Damon W: Some Do Care: Contemporary Lives of Moral Commitment. New York, Free Press, 1992

Coles R: The Moral Life of Children. Boston, MA, Atlantic Monthly Press, 1986

Coles R: Harvard Diary: Reflections on the Sacred and the Secular. New York, Crossroads, 1988

Coles R: The Moral Imagination of Children. New York, Random House, 1997

Comfort A: Directiveness in psychotherapy and the "sexual revolution." Psychiatry 44:318–326, 1981

Comte-Sponville A: A Small Treatise on the Great Virtues: The Uses of Philosophy in Everyday Life. New York, Henry Holt, 2001

Cooper A: Value systems and ego integration. Psychiatr Q 46:556–562, 1972

Costello RM: "Chicana Liberation" and the Mexican-American marriage. Psychiatric Annals 7:628–632, 1977

Crawshaw R, Rogers DE, Pellegrino ED, et al: Patient-physician covenant. JAMA 273:1553, 1995

Cushman P: Constructing the Self, Constructing America: A Cultural History of Psychotherapy. New York, Addison-Wesley, 1995

Damon W: Self-understanding and moral development from childhood to adolescence, in Morality, Moral Behavior and Moral Development. Edited by Kurtines W, Gewirtz J. New York, Wiley, 1984, pp 109–127

Damon W: The Moral Child: Nurturing Children's Natural Moral Growth. New York, Free Press, 1988

Damon W: Greater Expectations: Nurturing Children's Natural Moral Growth. New York, Free Press, 1995

Dawkins R: The Selfish Gene. Oxford, England, Oxford University Press, 1989

Dennett DC: Darwin's Dangerous Idea: Evolution and the Meanings of Life. New York, Simon & Schuster, 1995

de Waal F: Good Natured: The Origins of Right and Wrong in Humans and Other Animals. Cambridge, MA, Harvard University Press, 1996

Doherty WJ: Soul Searching: Why Psychotherapy Must Promote Moral Responsibility. New York, Basic Books, 1995

Dyer AR: The concept of character: moral and therapeutic considerations. Br J Med Psychol 59:35–41, 1986

Dyer AR: Ethics and Psychiatry: Toward Professional Definition. Washington, DC, American Psychiatric Press, 1988

Eisnitz AJ: On the metapsychology of narcissistic pathology. J Am Psychoanal Assoc 22:279–291, 1974

Emanuel EJ, Emanuel LL: Four models of the physician-patient relationship. JAMA 267:2221–2226, 1992

Engelhardt HT: Psychiatry as meta-ethics. Psychiatry 36:440–445, 1973

Finkelstein L: Neglected aspects of the superego. J Am Acad Psychoanal 19:530–554, 1991

Freud S: Mourning and melancholia (1917[1915]), in Standard Edition of the Complete Works of Sigmund Freud, Vol 14. Translated and edited by Strachey J. London, Hogarth Press, 1957, pp 237–260

Gartner J: The capacity to forgive: an object relations perspective. J Relig Health 27:313–318, 1988

Gilligan C: In a Different Voice: Psychological Theory and Women's Development. Cambridge, MA, Harvard University Press, 1993

Glueck S, Glueck E: Unraveling Juvenile Delinquency. New York, Commonwealth Fund, 1950

Goldberg C: The Evil We Do: The Psychoanalysis of Destructive People. Amherst, NY, Prometheus Books, 2000

Grand S: The Reproduction of Evil: A Clinical and Cultural Perspective. Hillsdale, NJ, Analytic Press, 2000

Greene JD, Somerville RB, Nystrom LE, et al: An fMRI investigation of emotional engagement in moral judgment. Science 293:2105–2108, 2001

Greenspan PS: Practical Guilt: Moral Dilemmas, Emotions and Social Norms. Oxford, England, Oxford University Press, 1995

Greifinger J: On the horizon of authenticity: toward a moral account of psychoanalytic theory, in Soul on the Couch: Spirituality, Religion and Morality in Contemporary Psychoanalysis. Edited by Spezzano C, Gargiulo GJ. Hillsdale, NJ, Analytic Press, 1997, pp 201–230

Gutheil TG: On the therapy in clinical administration, Parts I and II. Psychiatr Q 54:3–17, 1982

Halleck S: The Politics of Therapy. New York, Science House, 1971

Hamilton JW: Some cultural determinants of intrapsychic structure and psychopathology. Psychoanal Rev 58:223–244, 1971

Hargrave T: Families and Forgiveness: Healing Wounds in the Intergenerational Family. New York, Brunner/Mazel, 1994

Hauerwas S: A Community of Character: Toward a Constructive Christian Social Ethic. Notre Dame, IN, University of Notre Dame Press, 1981

Herman JL: Trauma and Recovery. New York, Basic Books, 1992

Higgins ET, Klein R, Strauman T: Self concept discrepancy theory: a psychological model for distinguishing among different aspects of depression and anxiety. Social Cognition 3:51–76, 1985

Higgins GO: Resilient Adults: Overcoming a Cruel Past. San Francisco, CA, Jossey-Bass, 1994

Hillman J, Ventura M: We've Had a Hundred Years of Psychotherapy—and the World's Getting Worse. San Francisco, CA, Harper San Francisco, 1992

Himmelfarb G: The De-moralization of Society. New York, Knopf, 1995

Hoffer A: Toward a definition of psychoanalytic neutrality. J Am Psychoanal Assoc 33:771–795, 1985

Holmes J, Lindley R: The Values of Psychotherapy. Oxford, England, Oxford University Press, 1989

Hope D: The healing power of forgiveness. Psychotherapy 24:240–244, 1987

Hundert EM: Lessons From an Optical Illusion: On Nature and Nurture, Knowledge and Values. Cambridge, MA, Harvard University Press, 1995

James W: The Varieties of Religious Experience (1903). New York, New American Library, 1958

Johnson A, Szurek S: The genesis of antisocial acting out in children and adolescents. Psychiatric Q 20:323–343, 1952

Johnson M: Moral Imagination: Implications of Cognitive Science for Ethics. Chicago, IL, University of Chicago Press, 1993

Jones LG: Transformed Judgment: Toward a Trinitarian Account of the Moral Life. Notre Dame, IN, University of Notre Dame Press, 1990

Jones LG: Embodying Forgiveness: A Theological Analysis. Grand Rapids, MI, WB Eerdmans, 1995

Jones S: A constructive relationship for religion with the science and profession of psychology: perhaps the boldest model yet. Am Psychol 49:184–199, 1994

Kagan J, Resnick JS, Clark C: Biological bases of childhood shyness. Science 240:167–171, 1988a

Kagan J, Resnick JS, Clark C, et al: Childhood derivatives of inhibition and lack of inhibition to the unfamiliar. Child Dev 55:2212–2225, 1988b

Kass LR: The Hungry Soul: Eating and the Perfecting of Our Nature. New York, Free Press, 1994

Kelly TA, Strupp HH: Patient and therapist values in psychotherapy: perceived changes, assimilation, similarity and outcome. J Consult Clin Psychol 60: 34–40, 1992

Kernberg OF: Object Relations Theory and Classical Psychoanalysis. New York, Jason Aronson, 1976

Kierkegaard S: Purity of Heart Is to Will One Thing (1847). New York, Harper & Brothers, 1938

Kierkegaard S: The Sickness Unto Death (1849). Princeton, NJ, Princeton University Press, 1968

Klein M: A contribution to the theory of anxiety and guilt. Int J Psychoanal 29:114–123, 1948

Kohlberg L: Essays in Moral Development, Vols 1 and 2: The Psychology of Moral Development. New York, Harper & Row, 1983

Kohlberg L, Ryncarz RA: Beyond justice reasoning: moral development and consideration of a seventh stage, in Higher Stages of Human Development: Perspectives on Adult Growth. Edited by Alexander CN, Langer EJ. New York, Oxford University Press, 1990, pp 191–207

Kovesi J: Moral Notions. London, Routledge & Kegan Paul, 1967

Kreitler H, Kreitler S: Cognitive Orientation and Behavior. New York, Springer, 1976

Kugler K, Jones WH: On conceptualizing and assessing guilt. J Pers Soc Psychol 62:318–327, 1992

Kultgen J: Autonomy and Intervention: Parentalism in the Caring Life. New York, Oxford University Press, 1995

Kurtines W, Gewirtz JL (eds): Morality, Moral Behavior, and Moral Development. New York, Wiley, 1984

Lagerman AG: The Moral Dimensions of Marriage and Family Therapy. Lanham, MD, University Press of America, 1993

Lakin M: Ethical Issues in the Psychotherapies. New York, Oxford University Press, 1988

Lakoff G: Moral Politics: What Conservatives Know That Liberals Don't. Chicago, IL, University of Chicago Press, 1996

Lakoff G, Johnson M: Metaphors We Live By. Chicago, IL, University of Chicago Press, 1980

Lamb S: The Trouble With Blame: Victims, Perpetrators and Responsibility. Cambridge, MA, Harvard University Press, 1996

Langmuir GI: Toward a Definition of Antisemitism. Berkeley, CA, University of California Press, 1990

Lax RF: The narcissistic investments in pathological character traits and the narcissistic depression: some implications for treatment. Int J Psychoanal 70:81–90, 1989

Levine S: The development of wickedness—from whence does evil stem? Psychiatr Ann 27:617–623, 1997

Lewis CS: The Abolition of Man. New York, Macmillan, 1947

Lewis CS: Studies in Words. London, Cambridge University Press, 1960

Lewis T, Amini F, Lannon R: A General Theory of Love. New York, Random House, 2000

Lifton RJ: Advocacy and corruption in the healing professions. Int Rev Psychoanal 3:409–415, 1976

London P: The Modes and Morals of Psychotherapy, 2nd Edition. New York, Holt, Rinehart & Winston, 1986

MacIntyre A: After Virtue, 2nd Edition. Notre Dame, IN, University of Notre Dame Press, 1984

Macklin R: Values in psychoanalysis and psychotherapy: a survey and analysis. Am J Psychoanal 33:133–150, 1973

Margalit A: The Ethics of Memory. Cambridge, MA, Harvard University Press, 2002

Margolis J: Psychotherapy and Morality: A Study of Two Concepts. New York, Random House, 1966

May R: Values, myths and symbols. Am J Psychiatry 132:703–706, 1975

McCullough ME, Pargament KI, Thoresen CE (eds): Forgiveness: Theory, Research and Practice. New York, Guilford, 2000

McGlashan TH, Miller GH: The goals of psychoanalysis and psychoanalytic psychotherapy. Arch Gen Psychiatry 39:377–388, 1982

Meloy JR: The Psychopathic Mind. New York, Jason Aronson, 1992

Milrod D: The ego ideal. Psychoanal Study Child 45:43–60, 1990

Miller JM: Toward a New Psychology of Women. Boston, MA, Beacon Press, 1976

Modell AH: On having the right to a life: an aspect of the superego's development. Int J Psychoanal 46:323–31, 1965

Mollinger RN: Antitheses and the obsessive-compulsive. Psychoanal Rev 67: 465–477, 1980

Morrison AP: Shame: The Underside of Narcissism. Hillsdale, NJ, Analytic Press, 1989

Mowrer OH: Morality and Mental Health. Chicago, IL, Rand-McNally, 1967

Mullan H: Inherent moral practice in group psychotherapy. Int J Group Psychotherapy 41:185–197, 1991

Mullen JD: Kierkegaard's Philosophy: Self-Deception and Cowardice in the Present Age. New York, The New American Library, 1981

Nicholas MW: The Mystery of Goodness and the Positive Moral Consequences of Psychotherapy. New York, WW Norton, 1994

Nucci LP: Challenging conventional wisdom about morality: the domain approach to values education, in Moral Development and Character Education: A Dialogue. Edited by Nucci LP. Berkeley, CA, McCutchan, 1989, pp 183–203

Nussbaum MC: Upheavals of Thought: The Intelligence of Emotions. Cambridge, England, Cambridge University Press, 2001

Olarte SW: Characteristics of therapists who become involved in sexual boundary violations. Psychiatric Annals 21:657–660, 1991

Overholser JC: Elements of the Socratic method, VI: promoting virtue in everyday life. Psychotherapy 36:137–145, 1999

Paredes J, Beyerstein D, Ledwidge B, et al: Psychiatric ethics and ethical psychiatry. Can J Psychiatry 35:600–603, 1990

Parekh B: Bentham's theory of virtue, in Can Virtue Be Taught? Edited by Darling-Smith B. Notre Dame, IN, University of Notre Dame Press, 1993, pp 53–68

Pattison EM: Morality, guilt, and forgiveness in psychotherapy, in Clinical Psychiatry and Religion. Edited by Pattison EM. Boston, MA, Little, Brown, 1969, pp 93–115

Pellegrino ED, Thomasma DC: The Christian Virtues in Medical Practice. Washington, DC, Georgetown University Press, 1996

Piaget J: The Moral Judgement of the Child (1932). Translated by Gabain M. New York, Free Press, 1965

Piers G, Singer MB: Shame and Guilt: A Psychoanalytic and a Cultural Inquiry. New York, WW Norton, 1971

Plantinga C: Not the Way It's Supposed to Be: A Breviary of Sin. Grand Rapids, MI, WB Eerdmans, 1995

Porter J: Moral Action and Christian Ethics. Cambridge, England, Cambridge University Press, 1995

Power FC, Higgins A, Kohlberg L: Lawrence Kohlberg's Approach to Moral Education. New York, Columbia University Press, 1989

Prosen M, Clark DC, Harrow M, et al: Guilt and conscience in major depressive disorders. Am J Psychiatry 140:839–844, 1983

Quay HC, Routh DK, Shapiro SK: Psychopathology of childhood: from description to validation. Ann Rev Psychol 38:491–532, 1987

Rabkin LY: Superego process in a collective society: the Israeli kibbutz. Int J Soc Psychiatry 21:79–86, 1975

Rapoport JL: The biology of obsessions and compulsions. Sci Am 260:82–89, 1989

Rawls J: A Theory of Justice. Cambridge, MA, Harvard University Press, 1971

Raynor JO, McFarlin DB: (1986) Motivation and the self-system, in Handbook of Motivation and Cognition: Foundations of Social Behavior. Edited by Sorrentino RM, Higgins ET. New York, Guilford, 1986, pp 315–349

Rest JR: The major components of morality, in Morality, Moral Behavior, and Moral Development. Edited by Kurtines WM, Gewirtz JL. New York, Wiley, 1984, pp 24–40

Rest JR: Moral Development: Advances in Research and Theory. New York, Praeger, 1986

Richards PS, Bergin AE: A Spiritual Strategy for Counseling and Psychotherapy. Washington, DC, American Psychological Association, 1997

Rieff P: Freud: The Mind of the Moralist. London, Methuen, 1959

Rieff P: The Triumph of the Therapeutic: Uses of Faith After Freud. New York, Harper & Row, 1966

Rozin P: Moralization, in Morality and Health. Edited by Brandt AM, Rozin P. New York, Routledge, 1997, pp 379–401

Ryan K, McLean G (eds): Character Education in Schools and Beyond. New York, Praeger, 1987

Samson R, Laub J: Crime in the Making: Pathways and Turning Points Through Life. Cambridge, MA, Harvard University Press, 1993

Schafer R: Retelling a Life: Narration and Dialogue in Psychoanalysis. New York, Basic Books, 1992

Schimmel S: Wounds Not Healed by Time: The Power of Repentance and Forgiveness. Oxford, England, Oxford University Press, 2002

Schonfeld WA: Adolescent turmoil and the search for identity. Am J Psychoanal 31:19–34, 1971

Schultz-Ross RA, Gutheil TG: Difficulties integrating spirituality into psychotherapy. J Psychother Pract Res 6:130–138, 1997

Schneider CE: The Practice of Autonomy: Patients, Doctors and Medical Decisions. Oxford, England, Oxford University Press, 1998

Sederer L: Moral therapy and the problem of morale. Am J Psychiatry 134:267–272, 1977

Segal H: Introduction to the Work of Melanie Klein, 2nd Edition. New York, Basic Books, 1974

Shaffer HJ: Denial, ambivalence and countertransference hate, in The Dynamics and Treatment of Alcoholism. Edited by Levin J, Weiss R. New York, Jason Aronson, 1994, pp 422–437

Sider RC: The ethics of therapeutic modality choice. Am J Psychiatry 141:390–394, 1984

Singer JL, Salovey P: Organized knowledge structures and personality: person schemas, self schemas, prototypes, and scripts, in Person Schemas and Maladaptive Interpersonal Patterns. Edited by Horowitz MJ. Chicago, IL, University of Chicago Press, 1991, pp 33–79

Singer M: Delinquency and family disciplinary configurations: an elaboration of the superego lacunae concept. Arch Gen Psychiatry 31:795–798, 1974

Slote M: From Morality to Virtue. Oxford, England, Oxford University Press, 1992

Smedes LB: Forgive and Forget: Healing the Hurts We Don't Deserve. New York, Simon & Schuster, 1984

Spiegel J: Transactions. New York, Science House, 1971

Stilwell BM, Galvin M, Kopta SM: Conceptualization of conscience in normal children and adolescents, ages 5 to 17. J Am Acad Child Adolesc Psychiatry 30:16–21, 1991

Stilwell BM, Galvin M, Kopta SM, et al: Moral-emotional responsiveness: a two-factor domain of conscience functioning. J Am Acad Child Adolesc Psychiatry 33:130–139, 1994

Stilwell BM, Galvin MR, Kopta SM, et al: Moral volition: the fifth and final domain leading to an integrated theory of conscience understanding. J Am Acad Child Adolesc Psychiatry 37:202–210, 1998

Stone AA: Law, Psychiatry, and Morality: Essays and Analysis. Washington, DC, American Psychiatric Press, 1984

Streng FJ, in Can Virtue Be Taught? Edited by Darling-Smith B. Notre Dame, IN, University of Notre Dame Press, 1993

Suess L, Halpern MS: Obsessive-compulsive disorder: the religious perspective, in Obsessive-Compulsive Disorder in Children and Adolescents. Edited by Rapoport JL. Washington, DC, American Psychiatric Press, 1989, pp 311–326

Szasz TS: Ideology and Insanity: Essays on the Psychiatric Dehumanization of Man. New York, M Boyars, 1983

Taylor C: Sources of the Self: The Making of the Modern Identity. Cambridge, MA, Harvard University Press, 1989

Tierney NL: Imagination and Ethical Ideals: Prospects for a Unified Philosophical and Psychological Understanding. Albany, State University of New York Press, 1994

Tjeltveit AC: The ethics of value conversion in psychotherapy: appropriate and inappropriate therapist influence on client values. Clin Psychol 6:515–537, 1986

Tjeltveit AC: Ethics and Values in Psychotherapy. London, Routledge, 1999

Tyson P, Tyson RL: Narcissism and superego development. J Am Psychoanal Assoc 32:75–98, 1984

Vaillant GE: Sociopathy as a human process. Arch Gen Psychiatry 32:178–183, 1975

Vaillant GE: Adaptation to Life. Boston, MA, Little, Brown, 1977

Veatch RM: Abandoning informed consent. Hastings Cent Rep 25:5–12, 1995

Viederman M, Perry SW: Use of a psychodynamic life narrative in the treatment of depression in the physically ill. Gen Hospital Psychiatry 3:177–185, 1980

Weiner NO: The Harmony of the Soul: Mental Health and Moral Virtue Reconsidered. Albany, State University of New York Press, 1993

Welner M: Defining evil: a depravity scale for today's courts. Forensic Echo 2:4–12, 1998

Will OA: Values and the psychotherapist. Am J Psychoanal 41:203–212, 1981

Wilson JQ: The Moral Sense. New York, Free Press, 1993

Worthey JA: The Ethics of the Ordinary in Healthcare: Concepts and Cases. Chicago, IL, Health Administration Press, 1997, pp 229–237

Worthington EL (ed): Dimensions of Forgiveness: Psychological Research and Theological Perspectives. Radnor, PA, Templeton Foundation Press, 1998

Wright R: The Moral Animal: Why We Are the Way We Are: The New Science of Evolutionary Psychology. New York, Random House, 1994

Wuthnow R: God and Mammon in America. New York, Free Press, 1994

Young-Bruehl E: The Anatomy of Prejudices. Cambridge, MA, Harvard University Press, 1996

CHAPTER
2

Shaping the Direction of Treatment

> The overcoming of resistances is the part of our work that requires the most time and the greatest trouble.
>
> *Sigmund Freud*

Patients, therapists, and third parties often bring differing values to the treatment situation. Traditionally trained psychotherapists generally encourage self-determination, whereas some patients value altruism to the point of self-defeating sacrifice, and some feminists place a higher priority on relatedness. Many individuals object to the idea of dependence on medication to feel less distressed. Parents may well want certain outcomes that their child who is in treatment does not. Insurance companies value efficiency.

Clinicians rarely discuss explicitly how such competing value commitments should influence the direction of a patient's treatment. Most would agree that the patient-clinician relationship should be collaborative or deliberative rather than simply informative or paternalistic (Balint and Shelton 1996; Emanuel and Emanuel 1992; Sider 1984). However, mental health professionals lack a common understanding of what this means in practical terms. This chapter considers the relevance of moral decision making (cf. Chapter 1) in planning a course of treatment (Figure 2). It highlights the moral questions involved and lays out a general approach to them rather than attempting to answer each one.

Evaluating the Situation, Including Its Value Dimensions

At first glance, it may seem easy for clinicians to objectively assess the factors important in planning a course of treatment. Patient characteristics (e.g., presenting problem, probable diagnosis, character traits, premorbid adjustment, family situation, and willingness to consider one approach vs. another), the evidence for the effectiveness of possible treatments, and the availability of resources.

Yet biased or deficient assessment of the patient's characteristics regularly contributes to negative outcomes (Hadley and Strupp 1976). Because clinicians' value preferences influence what they see, patients often receive the treatments their clinicians know best rather than those that are most effective (Talbott 1990). For example, a "here and now" marital treatment may founder because of inattention to the intractable intrapsychic conflicts of one spouse (Kluft 1992). A behavior therapist may neglect problems raised by the transferential aspect of her techniques. An individual therapist may fail to appreciate the implications of the therapy for the patient's marriage. A psychoanalyst treating a narcissistic woman who is psychologically abusive to her children may fail to insist on intervention on the children's behalf. A family therapist eager to rehabilitate a dysfunctional family may not adequately address the needs of a daughter who has suffered incest and who may be better served by being removed from that family. In the case of *Osherhoff v. Chestnut Lodge*, monetary damages resulted from the failure of a psychodynamically oriented hospital staff to use accepted somatic means in treating a major depression (Klerman 1990). On the other hand, overdiagnosis of medication-responsive conditions has become all too common (Baldessarini 2000).

> A 40-year-old building superintendent requested medication for anxiety, restlessness, and difficulty concentrating. His girlfriend accompanied him to explain her conviction that these symptoms and the tension in their relationship were due to an undiagnosed "chemical imbalance."

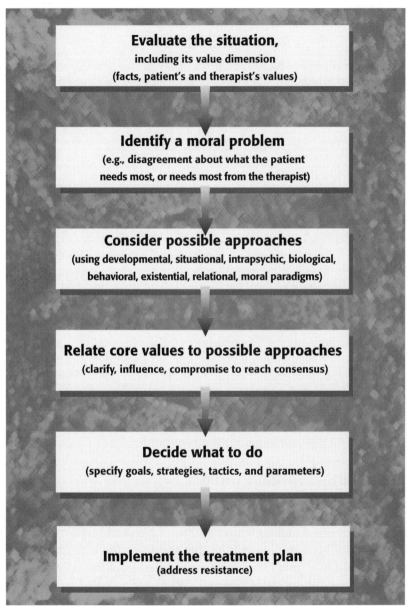

FIGURE 2. Steps of moral decision making in treatment planning.

A research-oriented psychiatrist they saw diagnosed an atypical bipolar disorder and offered the patient participation in a medication trial that she was conducting. After several weeks, when the patient felt sedated but no better taking valproic acid, he sought another opinion.

A second psychiatrist focused on several unresolved problems in the patient's life, including a recent conviction for sexually abusing his

daughter, a subsequent divorce with loss of visitation rights, and growing expectations of his new girlfriend. The patient resisted his recom-
mendation of psychotherapy but agreed to a brief trial of Ritalin for a
possible diagnosis of attention-deficit/hyperactivity disorder. When this
failed, his girlfriend helped him find a third psychiatrist who prescribed
antianxiety medication for a time before he dropped out of treatment.

In this case, the research psychopharmacologist's support for a medication solution diverted the attention of the patient and his girlfriend from
other equally important elements of the case.

There are other potential sources of bias in assessment. Role-related
assumptions can lead clinicians to formulate the same case in different
ways (Lazare 1973). A physician might focus on diagnosable disorders;
a psychological expert, on problematic dynamics or behaviors; and a social worker, on the adequacy of family and other support. Psychotherapeutic schools have their own diagnostic preferences (Lakin 1988; London 1986; Ratzinger 1998; Stone 1984).

In addition to the facts of the case and these potential sources of bias
stemming from their own values, clinicians clearly must assess what
matters most to the patient and what changes he expects the therapy to
bring about.

Finally, the agendas of involved third parties deserve attention. If
parents are paying for a child's care, what are the parents' concerns? How
involved do they expect to be in the treatment? What is the influence of
a managed care company or a government regulator on services offered? What is a pharmaceutical company hoping to gain by providing a
clinician with educational or research support?

Identifying a Moral Problem

Despite differences in how they see the problem, patients and therapists
usually reach an implicit consensus on a shared set of goals for their
work together. Exceptions of three types present moral obstacles to the
process of treatment planning.

The first is difficulty *knowing what is best for the patient*. Would a
trauma survivor with borderline features benefit most from symptom
relief, insight, relatedness, behavioral control, or growth? Prioritizing these requires a clinician to weigh several possible conceptions of
health.

A second related difficulty is *deciding what role the therapist should
play in the patient's life*. Is it best for the clinician to serve as consultant,
supportive advocate, insight-oriented or cognitive-behavioral therapist, administrator, or medication backup? If a clinician wants to play

only a limited role in the life of a potentially demanding patient, is this fair to a patient who may lack access to equally good treatment options? When is the therapist justified in addressing problems that concern her more than the patient?

A 20-year-old college student with active substance abuse, a history of depression, and a chaotic family background discussed with her therapist the possibility of working as a strip dancer and making extra money by installing Internet cameras in her bathroom. Her therapist explored her motivations but wondered if his role should include expressing concerns about whether these might not be good choices for her.

A third moral difficulty in planning treatment is *frank disagreement about the direction of the work*. (Framing the problem this way is not meant to imply that a therapist and patient necessarily occupy a level playing field; the power differential that characterizes therapy also raises important moral issues.) Somatically oriented patients often want psychopharmacology to play a larger role in their treatment than do their clinicians, whereas depressed or paranoid patients may resist taking medication. Patients with borderline personality disorder may insist that they need more individual attention from therapists, who may instead believe they need limits, additional outside support, or exploration of their feelings. Abusive or narcissistic patients may not agree with their therapists about the fact that there are prosocial values that are essential for them to acquire.

Considering Possible Courses of Action

In the face of uncertainty about the best course of action, clinicians must consider a full range of therapeutic models or paradigms (Lazare 1973; Perry et al. 1990; Yager 1977).

1. A *developmental* paradigm focuses on successful transitions between life stages—for example, the achievement of identity by an adolescent or of Eriksonian integrity by an older adult.
2. A *situational* paradigm recognizes the important impact of a loss such as a death, illness, or divorce.
3. A *biological* paradigm, already established in the treatment of major mental illnesses, is now being invoked in the treatment of anxiety, depression, and even undesirable personality traits (Kramer 1993).
4. *Cognitive* and *behavioral* paradigms frame approaches to the habitual components of conditions that range from anxiety and depression to personality disorders (Beck 1976, 1990). For example, limit setting

and reinforcement of alternative behaviors (as in dialectical behavior therapy) have become central to the treatment of deliberate self-harm in patients with borderline personality disorder.

5. Therapists use an *intrapsychic* paradigm to help patients resolve repressed and/or unresolved emotional conflicts, such as an oedipal work inhibition or object choice. Their techniques for increasing patients' insight and mastery include clarification, confrontation, interpretation, encouragement to elaborate, empathic validation, and affirmation (Gabbard 2000; Makover 1996).

6. A *relational* paradigm emphasizes helping patients to function within an interpersonal context with greater empathy, communication, and concern. Pioneers in bringing a relational perspective into the psychotherapeutic process include Harry Stack Sullivan, object relations theorists such as Fairbairn, family therapists such as Minuchin, general systems theorists such as Bertalanffy, and feminist clinicians such as Gilligan. A systems perspective might be important for stabilizing a family crisis.

7. An *existential* paradigm recognizes that patients often struggle with inescapable conditions such as death anxiety, the search for meaning, and the need to make basic choices in life (Baumeister 1991; Yalom 1980). Helping a dying patient reach acceptance and a sense of purpose (Weisman 1993) might include helping him to resolve a religious or spiritual problem.[1]

8. A clinician might use a *moral* paradigm to help his patient clarify and integrate her moral commitments, use these commitments to make moral decisions, address obstacles to implementing these commitments (e.g., an addiction), accurately assess responsibilities and failures (establish realistic guilt), deal effectively with moral failures (both in herself and in others), and develop morally admirable (virtuous) character traits.

Relating Values to Possible Courses of Action

We considered earlier the need to recognize biases that can distort diagnostic assessment. Just as they must recognize the influence of cul-

---

[1]DSM-IV-TR (American Psychiatric Association 2000, p. 741) defines religious or spiritual problems, using a V code, as "distressing experiences that involve loss or questioning of faith, problems associated with conversion to a new faith, or questioning of spiritual values that may not necessarily be related to an organized church or religious institution."

tural or countertransferential factors, clinicians must identify the values that guide their choice of a treatment paradigm. Most clinicians embrace the ideals of autonomy/freedom to choose, adaptability/flexibility, and the ability to function in important areas such as love and work (cf. Freud). Many also join feminists in making relatedness an important goal (Miller 1976). Evidence is increasingly available for assessing the effectiveness of various therapeutic approaches in achieving these aims. However, because clinicians rarely make explicit their conceptions of mental health (Havens 1984; Vaillant 2003), they often fail to see how they inevitably give various ideals different relative weight. A clinician who values individual autonomy more than connectedness to others will tend to favor an intrapsychic over a relational approach. One who values symptom-free functioning over self-knowledge is likely to favor a biological or a behavioral over an intrapsychic strategy. One who values moral and spiritual functioning will be more likely to consider whether problems in giving and finding forgiveness are both causes and effects of his patient's problems. A therapist who sees morality and religion as reducible to psychodynamic processes will tend to give relatively less importance to a patient's struggles with a supreme being.

How can therapists respectfully take a patient's values into account while presenting a vision for change? Of the three common ways of influencing patients—explanation, persuasion, and negotiation—explanation is the least coercive. Richards and Bergin (1997, p. 125) explain their use of a spiritual paradigm to patients as follows:

> My orientation as a counselor is "eclectic." In selecting treatment methods, therefore, I tend to draw on ideas and techniques from a number of the major counseling approaches whose utility has been supported through research (e.g., cognitive therapy, behavioral therapy, client-centered therapy, family systems therapy, and psychodynamic therapy). I also believe that a spiritual perspective is important in counseling, and I am open to exploring any religious or spiritual concerns or issues you may have. I may also suggest that you participate in spiritual practices or interventions that are compatible with your beliefs if I believe they may help in your growth and progress. Of course, you will never be compelled to participate in psychological or spiritual interventions that you do not wish to engage in.

Explanation may stimulate discussion based on a patient's reflection and reading of the professional literature, direct pharmaceutical advertising, or material culled from the Internet.

At times clinicians also must persuade patients to accept what they believe is in their best interest (e.g., treatment with antipsychotic medication) using an empathic understanding of the patient to establish a working alliance (Margulies and Havens 1981): "I know that your independence and caring for your family are very important to you. My concern, based on your history, is that failing to take medication will put you at serious risk of relapsing and returning to the hospital."

When persuasion fails, there may be a need for negotiation and compromise. A psychiatrist might agree to discontinue medication if the patient agrees to resume taking it at the first sign of a recurrence of symptoms.

When a clinician and her patient fail to come together on important values and a paradigm for treatment, the clinician may either acknowledge that too little agreement exists or insist on involuntary treatment if she judges her patient to be in danger (Group for the Advancement of Psychiatry 1994; Kultgen 1995). Deciding when a patient is in serious enough danger to warrant commitment involves carefully balancing the patient's rights and the clinician's responsibilities.

Deciding What to Do

Agreement between patient and therapist on overall ideals, aims, and approaches is not enough (Sadler and Hulgus 1992); good treatment planning is also pragmatic and specific. One benefit of managed care has been to challenge clinicians to think through the relationship between their treatment aims (operationalized by reviewers as desired outcomes) and the goals, strategies, tactics, and parameters of the work. Goals define the intermediate conditions necessary to achieve therapeutic aims; in a depressed patient, they might include a reduction in symptoms and greater involvement with others (Makover 1996). Strategies constitute specific treatment modalities selected to achieve goals, such as psychodynamic psychotherapy, behavior modification, or pharmacotherapy. The technical elements used to pursue these strategies are tactics such as interpretation, desensitization, or neuroleptic medication. Strategies and tactics help to specify the parameters of treatment, such as setting (office, hospital, etc.), format (individual, group, etc.), and time (length and frequency of sessions and duration of treatment) (Perry et al. 1990).

Specifying these conditions of treatment helps clinicians make interventions more evidence-based. It also helps them to recognize when disagreements (e.g., with patients or managed care reviewers) over goals, strategies, or tactics actually reflect more fundamental differences in aims (e.g., symptom relief, behavioral change, or growth).

Implementing a Treatment Plan

Both therapist- and patient-related obstacles can hinder implementation of an agreed-upon treatment plan. Therapist-related obstacles include financial disincentives; countertransference-based wishes to please or to control; and everyday factors such as anxiety, fatigue, restlessness, and simple inattentiveness (Nicholi 1999). Overcoming such obstacles requires professional virtues such as patience, courage, and integrity, nurtured by the support and guidance of others (Chapter 1).

Patient-related obstacles can be primarily cognitive, affective, relational, or moral. *Cognitive* obstacles represent misapprehensions about the central problem or the nature of the treatment (Beck 1976, 1990). For example, a patient might believe he could become physically dependent on an antidepressant or that his condition would become worse if he explored a painful loss. Therapists may need to confront ingrained cognitive distortions such as rationalization or other maladaptive schemas (Horowitz 1991) through the use of cognitive strategies such as reframing, guided discovery, or deliberate exaggeration (see Beck 1976, 1990).

Insight is rarely enough to help a patient relinquish maladaptive patterns, and clinicians often must address *affective* resistance to treatment. By empathizing with the anxiety and other painful affects associated with the loss of these patterns, she can help her patient bear them and tolerate the impact of needed confrontation, interpretation, or clarification ("giving with one hand while taking with the other"). When a therapist's supportive contribution is not enough and the pain associated with therapeutic change becomes intolerable to the patient, the therapist may also need to enlist the support of medication, family members, or a group.

A patient's *relational* or transferential resistance (e.g., a passive-aggressive style) may have to become a central focus (Stark 1994). Therapists can sometimes help a patient to "restructure" characterological resistance by relinquishing maladaptive defenses, learning more adaptive ones, and reconfiguring representations of himself and others (Vaillant 1997).

Moral obstacles to treatment can overlap with these categories of resistance but are also usefully considered in their own right. A patient may be unsure what is right for him to do, reluctant to change because of guilt or shame, too resentful to consider forgiving a spouse, prone to acting destructively, or lacking in empathy. The rest of this chapter explores several forms of moral resistance and ways of addressing them using a moral paradigm.

Moral Reservations

How should one approach a patient's concern that it is wrong to take an antidepressant because it means "depending on a medicine to deal with life's problems?" What does this conviction suggest about the patient's moral functioning? Is she depending uncritically for guidance on something a religious leader has taught, or has she always believed in the importance of learning from suffering? Has depression made her unable to reason clearly about her best interests? To the extent that the patient has realistic moral reservations, a therapist would want to help the patient clarify her sources of moral authority and use them to reason through her dilemmas (Chapter 1).

Guilt and Shame

If the patient feels undeserving of a therapist's help, is this because he never has valued himself? Does he lack a way to deal with real moral failure? Is his capacity to assess his shortcomings distorted by depression?

> A 40-year-old nurse came for treatment at her supervisor's insistence. She described long-standing moderate depression marked by limited enjoyment, intermittent alcohol abuse, and social isolation. Working long hours helped her to feel she was both doing something worthwhile for someone else and being suitably punished for an affair and subsequent divorce.
>
> After antidepressants lifted her mood somewhat, she began to consider why it had always been so difficult for her to enjoy herself. What emerged was that her critical and devaluing mother had assigned her to care for seven younger siblings with few resources. She had never felt entitled to have more, even as an adult.

This patient's therapist addressed the patient's shame by asking her to suspend judgment long enough to understand why she felt so burdened. Insight into her tendency to assess herself too harshly helped the patient both to accept treatment and to allow herself more pleasure in life.

Patients sometimes become caught up in a compulsive cycle of guilt, self-recrimination, rationalization, and reinvolvement in self-destructive activities (e.g., substance abuse, gambling, or pornography).

> While actively abusing cocaine and alcohol, a 30-year-old man stole to support his habit and neglected to use sterile needles. However, when not "just wanting to get high," he felt guilt over his behavior, which served as a reason to escape into further drug use. His drug counselor

both pointed out his potential for losing his better judgment with his next drug high and encouraged him to find an effective way of dealing with guilt.

This patient moved forward only after beginning to practice the fourth and fifth steps of Alcoholics Anonymous: taking a "fearless and searching moral inventory" and confessing his wrongs to another person. Many individuals experience guilt or shame in religious terms. Although some conservative patients mistrust therapists who do not share their worldview, such clinicians can often help patients with religiously reinforced guilt to understand whether their reading of their tradition is accurate and to consider the avenues it provides for forgiveness, or they can refer these patients to other resources such as a pastoral counselor (Bollinger 1985; Peteet 1994; Probst et al. 1992).

Moralism

Idealism sometimes takes the form of problematic scrupulosity in obsessional and perfectionistic patients.

> A graduate student felt angry and depressed after slights by friends and professors whom she had expected to be more consistent and careful. Exploration revealed an exaggerated sense of fairness that led to repeated disappointment both in others and in herself. In working to help her develop more realistic expectations, her therapist proceeded cautiously, aware that he could lose her trust if he undermined her idealism.

More disturbed individuals use primitive defenses of splitting and projection to devalue and idealize others. They may need help to recognize the all-or-nothing distortions that characterize their thinking and to develop a greater capacity for forgiveness toward themselves and others (Gartner 1988; Schafer 1992; Stark 1994).

> A 50-year-old musician came for treatment because of depression and rage toward a growing list of physicians. She complained that some had patronized her during treatment for colon cancer and that others had missed diagnoses of hypothyroidism, allergic asthma, and fibroids. Resentful that they could discount her complaints because they were more powerful and "could just get away with it," she seemed entrenched in the role of victim and preoccupied with "making them pay."
>
> Her therapist tried unsuccessfully to help her see what she might have contributed to these ill-fated encounters with physicians. He also tried pointing out how her feelings toward the physicians resembled the bitterness and indignation she felt toward her estranged parents, whom she described as tyrannical and devaluing. She saw the parallel but felt little helped.

On several occasions, she criticized her therapist for his own inattentiveness to her complaints but forgave him when he apologized, acknowledging that he had listened patiently to most of them. Over time, she began to show a similarly compassionate, more realistic assessment of some of her other caretakers. Eventually, she focused less on others and more on how her unforgiving attitude toward herself interfered with her ability to perform.

This patient's sensitivity to being wronged almost aborted her psychotherapy, just as it had many other episodes of medical care. Initially lacking in strategies to deal with the moral failings of others, she used her relationship with a normal, imperfect therapist to acquire some and to become more forgiving. In an important sense, the treatment of this woman's personality disorder was a moral intervention.

Narcissism

The narcissism of many patients with borderline and antisocial personality disorders sometimes requires that the patient be confronted to achieve meaningful change.

A 35-year-old lawyer came for treatment because of unsatisfying relationships with men. She felt excited by the challenge of securing a new man's attention but typically lost interest and moved on to someone else. Initially appreciative of her male therapist, she began to miss sessions with him without notice. Her therapist concluded that narcissistic and histrionic traits were responsible for her superficial and exploitative relationships and confronted her failure of empathy by asking if she had considered the feelings of the men she had left. After her initial shock at the question, she began to appreciate what had interfered with achieving her goal of a longer-lasting and more satisfying relationship.

Patients with character disorders such as those whom Freeman and Gunderson (1989) described as having disorders of the "core self" typically require external input to experience and deal with guilt in normal ways (Vaillant 1975). Effective value-laden (moral) input may come from influential individuals (Viederman 1986), a highly structured cognitive-behavioral group treatment (Linehan 1993), or a 12-step program.

The treatment of narcissistic individuals with antisocial traits presents special moral challenges. These individuals may lack not only empathy but also sufficient integrity, loyalty, or truthfulness to form a traditional therapeutic alliance (Meloy 1992; Reid et al. 1986; Stone 1993). When dangerous, they create moral as well as legal duties to warn their potential victims. So long as some severely antisocial individuals are at liberty, it may be unethical to provide treatment that seems likely to make them more successful at activities that harm others, such as drug dealing or money laundering (Goldberg 2000).

Traditionally, therapists have been more comfortable addressing problems involving excessive guilt (e.g., via a rational appeal to their self-identified goals or self-interest) than failures of empathy or responsibility (Doherty 1995). For example, Lovinger (1985) described only belatedly confronting his patient's superego lacuna when he recognized that their rational discussion in psychotherapy of the patient's leaving his wife and children had served as a defense against his patient's deeper conflictual feelings.

Masochism

Patients with prominent self-defeating or masochistic traits are notoriously resistant to treatment. Freud (1924) used the term *moral masochism* to denote the unconscious guilt he saw behind the tendency of these patients to accept and even seek roles in interpersonal situations that bring them significant adverse consequences. Martha Stark (1994) and others have focused on the role of poorly integrated aggression in the form of "triumphant autonomy" or "relentless entitlement" that often underlies such patients' apparent kindness, solicitude, politeness, and humility (Kernberg 1988; Parkin 1980). When a patient's religious belief system and/or community sanctions self-sacrifice or uncritically discourages aggression (Schwartz et al. 2001), clinicians may need to help them to think through what moral commitments are really their own. This may include enlisting resources such as a pastor, religious friends, or even reading of helpful scriptures and commentaries (Peteet 1994).

How, then, is it useful to think about treatment planning as a moral process and to address these forms of resistance in moral terms? For one thing, adopting a moral paradigm takes the patient's moral concerns seriously. For another, approaching these concerns as problems in moral functioning offers a structure for formulating specific moral interventions. Third, following the steps of moral reasoning gives the therapist a chance to articulate and legitimize the values she brings to treatment.

Conclusion

Patients, therapists, and third parties all contribute to shaping the direction of treatment. As we have seen, there are a number of moral aspects to this process at each step—assessment, recognition of conflicts, consideration of possible paradigms, application of therapeutic values to the selection of a specific approach, and implementation in the face of resistance can all be moral in nature. Making this process more explicit and shared helps to guard against overuse of a favored paradigm, including a moral one. It also makes the implications of value differences clearer. Subsequent chapters consider junctures in treatment where problems in moral functioning emerge that require clinician and patient to reassess the direction of their work in a similar way.

References

American Psychiatric Association: Diagnostic and Statistical Manual of Mental Disorders, 4th Edition, Text Revision. Washington, DC, American Psychiatric Association, 2000

Baldessarini RJ: A plea for the integrity of the bipolar disorder concept. Bipolar Disorders 2:3–7, 2000

Balint J, Shelton W: Regaining the initiative: forging a new model of the patient-physician relationship. JAMA 275:887–891, 1996

Baumeister RF: Meanings of Life. New York, Guilford, 1991

Beck AT: Cognitive Therapy and the Emotional Disorders. New York, International Universities Press, 1976

Beck AT, Freeman A, and associates: Cognitive Therapy of Personality Disorders. New York, Guilford, 1990

Bollinger RA: Differences between pastoral counseling and psychotherapy. Bull Menninger Clin 49:371–386, 1985

Doherty WJ: Soul Searching: Why Psychotherapy Must Promote Moral Responsibility. New York, Basic Books, 1995

Emanuel EJ, Emanuel LL: Four models of the physician-patient relationship. JAMA 267:2221–2226, 1992

Freeman PS, Gunderson SG: Treatment of personality disorders. Psychiatric Annals 19:147–153, 1989

Freud S: The economic problem of masochism (1924), in Standard Edition of the Complete Psychological Works of Sigmund Freud, Vol 19. Edited by Strachey J. London, Hogarth Press, 1974, pp 159–170

Gabbard GO: Psychodynamic Psychotherapy in Clinical Practice, 3rd Edition. Washington, DC, American Psychiatric Press, 2000

Gartner J: The capacity to forgive: an object relations perspective. J Relig Health 27:313–318, 1988

Goldberg C: The Evil We Do: The Psychoanalysis of Destructive People. Amherst, NY, Prometheus Books, 2000

Group for the Advancement of Psychiatry, Committee on Government Policy: Forced Into Treatment (GAP Report 137). Washington, DC, American Psychiatric Press, 1994

Hadley SW, Strupp HH: Contemporary views of negative effects in psychotherapy: an integrated account. Am J Psychiatry 33:1291–1302, 1976

Havens LL: The need for tests of normal functioning in the psychiatric interview. Am J Psychiatry 141:1208–1211, 1984

Horowitz MJ (ed): Person Schemas and Maladaptive Interpersonal Patterns. Chicago, IL, University of Chicago Press, 1991

Kernberg OF: Clinical dimensions of masochism. J Am Psychoanal Assoc 36:1005–1029, 1988

Klerman GL: The psychiatric patient's right to treatment: implications of *Osherhoff v Chestnut Lodge*. Am J Psychiatry 147:409–418, 1990

Kluft RP: Paradigm exhaustion and paradigm shift—thinking through the therapeutic impasse. Psychiatric Annals 22:502–508, 1992

Kramer PD: Listening to Prozac. New York, Viking, 1993

Kultgen J: Autonomy and Intervention: Parentalism in the Caring Life. New York, Oxford University Press, 1995

Lakin M: Ethical Issues in the Psychotherapies. New York, Oxford University Press, 1988

Lazare A: Hidden conceptual models in clinical psychiatry. New Engl J Med 288:345–354, 1973

Linehan MM: Cognitive-Behavioral Treatment of Borderline Personality Disorder. New York, Guilford, 1993

London P: The Modes and Morals of Psychotherapy, 2nd Edition. New York, Holt, Rinehart & Winston, 1986

Lovinger RJ: Religious imagery in the psychotherapy of a borderline patient, in Psychotherapy of the Religious Patient. Edited by Spero MH. Springfield, IL, Charles C Thomas, 1985, pp 181–205

Makover RB: Treatment Planning for Psychotherapists, 2nd Edition. Washington, DC, American Psychiatric Publishing, 2004

Margulies A, Havens LL: The initial encounter: what to do first? Am J Psychiatry 138:421–428, 1981

Meloy JR: The Psychopathic Mind: Origins, Dynamics, and Treatment. Northvale, NJ, Jason Aronson, 1992

Miller JM: Toward a New Psychology of Women. Boston, MA, Beacon Press, 1976

Nicholi A (ed): The Harvard Guide to Psychiatry. Cambridge, MA, Harvard University Press, 1999

Parkin A: On masochistic enthrallment: a contribution to the study of moral masochism. Int J Psychoanal 61:307–314, 1980

Perry S, Frances A, Clarkin J: DSM-III-R Casebook of Treatment Selection. New York, Brunner/Mazel, 1990

Peteet JR: Approaching spiritual problems in psychotherapy: a conceptual framework. J Psychother Pract Res 3:237–245, 1994

Probst LR, Ostrom R, Watkins P, et al: Comparative efficacy of religious and nonreligious cognitive therapy for the treatment of depression in religious individuals. J Consult Clin Psychol 60:94–103, 1992

Ratzinger SM: Shame in the therapeutic relationship, in Shame: Interpersonal Behavior, Psychopathology, and Culture. Edited by Gilbert P, Andrews B. New York, Oxford University Press, 1998, pp 206–222

Reid WH, Dorr D, Walker J, Bonner J: Unmasking the Psychopath. New York, WW Norton, 1986

Richards PS, Bergin AE: A Spiritual Strategy for Counseling and Psychotherapy. Washington, DC, American Psychological Association, 1997

Sadler JZ, Hulgus YF: Clinical problem solving and the biopsychosocial model. Am J Psychiatry 149:1315–1323, 1992

Schafer R: Retelling a Life: Narration and Dialogue in Psychoanalysis. New York, Basic Books, 1992

Sider R: The ethics of therapeutic modality choice. Am J Psychiatry 141:390–394, 1984

Stark M: Working With Resistance. Northvale, NJ, Jason Aronson, 1994

Stone AA: Law, Psychiatry, and Morality. Washington, DC, American Psychiatric Press, 1984

Stone MH: Abnormalities of Personality: Within and Beyond the Realm of Treatment. New York, WW Norton, 1993

Schwartz AC, Calhoun AW, Eschbach CL, et al: Treatment of conversion disorder in an African American Christian woman: cultural and social considerations. Am J Psychiatry 158:1385–1391, 2001

Talbott J: Foreword, in DSM-III-R Casebook of Treatment Selection. Edited by Perry S. Frances A, Clarkin J. New York, Brunner/Mazel, 1990, p xiv

Vaillant GE: Sociopathy as a human process. Arch Gen Psychiatry 32:178–183, 1975

Vaillant GE: Adaptation to Life. Boston, MA, Little, Brown, 1977

Vaillant GE: Mental health. Am J Psychiatry 160:1373–1384, 2003

Vaillant LM: Changing Character: Short-Term Anxiety-Regulating Psychotherapy for Restructuring Defenses, Affects and Attachment. New York, Basic Books, 1997

Viederman M: Personality change through life experience (I): a model. Psychiatry 49:204–217, 1986

Weisman AD: The Vulnerable Self: Confronting the Ultimate Questions. New York, Plenum, 1993

Yager J: Psychiatric eclecticism: a cognitive view. Am J Psychiatry 134:736–741, 1977

Yalom ID: Existential Psychotherapy. New York, Basic Books, 1980

CHAPTER 3

Caring for Patients

The secret of the care of the patient is in caring for the patient.

Francis Peabody, M.D.

You've got to love your patients.

Elvin Semrad, M.D.

Caring for vulnerable human beings is central to being a clinician, but what does it mean to care? How can we understand our failures and those of our colleagues to care effectively? How can we help trainees who harm or offend patients? We can best answer these questions if we come to understand caring as a moral activity.

As Dr. Peabody's dictum suggests, the term *care* has more than one meaning. To care can mean to *feel* toward others empathy, concern, or compassion (Branch 2000). It also can mean to *commit oneself* to achieving their best interests. Doing so in a caring fashion is to *behave in a nurturing fashion*—by tending to their needs. *Taking care* can also mean to *attend diligently* to these needs. This chapter considers briefly each of these meanings but finds them ultimately limited as guides to practice. It then traces the roots of these interrelated aspects of caring and correlates them to the moral development and functioning of clinicians.

Caring as Feeling

Growing attention to efficiency and technical expertise in medicine has prompted concern over the loss of the clinician's "human touch" (Cluff and Binstock 2001). Renewed interest in the clinician-patient relationship has focused on promoting compassionate care—for example, through teaching physicians empathic communication (Novack et al. 1997; Reich 1989; Schwartz 1995; Spiro 1995; Suchman et al. 1997). The use of the word *love* by psychiatrist Elvin Semrad (Rako and Mazur 1980) and primary care physician Eric Cassell (1997) underscores the emotional component of a clinician's empathic response to a patient.

Yet an affective approach to clinical care raises challenging questions. What makes it possible to experience fellow feelings toward patients? How much should clinicians feel? How can they feel strongly while also preserving their judgment, meeting their own needs, and avoiding burnout?

Caring as Commitment

Care can also mean taking responsibility for promoting a vulnerable patient's well-being. The Patient-Physician Covenant (Crawshaw 1995) reminds physicians that they are "both intellectually and morally obligated to act as advocates for the sick wherever their welfare is threatened and for their health at all times. . . . A recent Call to Action by the Ad Hoc Committee to Defend Health Care similarly highlights the duties of clinicians to relieve suffering, prevent and treat illness, and promote health ("For Our Patients, Not for Profits" 1997).

Clinicians are obligated to give their patients' needs priority in relation to competing economic, research, institutional, or ideological interests. Pellegrino and Thomasma (1997) have emphasized this point in relation to recent financial assaults and market paradigm pressures on clinicians working within the U.S. health care system. However, an understanding of caring as duty cannot by itself show clinicians how to care or how better to support caring.

Caring as Nurturing Behavior

Some have tried to conceptualize caring in behavioral, even measurable, terms. For example, several nursing investigators have developed standardized scales for assessing the frequency of behaviors patients and/or clinicians experience as caring, including an empathetic manner, continuity of presence, listening, and professional knowledge and skill (Andrews et al. 1996; Watson and Lea 1997). Callahan (2001) has described different levels of caring directed at patients' cognitive, emotional, value and relational needs. Researchers at Jefferson Medical College (Hojat et al. 2002) have developed a tool for measuring both affective and cognitive domains of physician empathy. Yet clinicians show caring behaviors because they care, not because these behaviors have been identified through research. Clinicians may learn from such behavioral research how to care more effectively, but not to care in the first place.

Caring as Diligence

A fourth traditional meaning of *care* is *diligent attention to quality*. At the beginning of the twentieth century, the Flexner Report on U.S. medical education sought to improve care by increasing the scrutiny given to undergraduate medical education. Health care professions subsequently instituted standardized examinations, licensing, certification, and continuing education. Quality assurance and improvement processes now include credentialing, accreditation, periodic reviews, practice guidelines, outcomes research, and evidence-driven practices. Leaders in health care delivery are considering ways to prevent errors by reducing reliance on memory, improving information access, computerizing standard protocols, and training clinicians in the operation of safe systems (Leape 1994). Yet a focus on regulatory details can also compete with a focus on the patient as a whole person. As a result, care as diligence offers only a partial perspective on what it means to care.

Caring as a Moral Activity

Understanding caring as a moral activity offers a more useful framework for addressing problems in caring than any one of the four meanings outlined above. Caring is integrally related to one's moral functioning. Early moral emotions such as sympathy shape one's commitments, including one's beliefs about what matters most (Chapter 1). Requisite virtues such as compassion and responsibility are sustained and shaped through experiences with others. They inform a prospective clinician's ideal self and may contribute to the choice of a profession that offers opportunity to nurture and to attend diligently to the needs of others. Consider how this perspective links and sheds light on various problems in caring.

Compassion

Compassion, or suffering with someone else, depends on empathy or accurately perceiving what he feels. It also involves identifying with the patient's best interests. The inability to respond compassionately lies at the root of many clinicians' problems in caring effectively.

> A 30-year-old surgical resident was suspended from his program because of complaints about his insensitive and offensive behavior. He recalled being "a bit overbearing" in medical school but felt he had functioned well as an intern and was very distressed to learn that a series of incidents had threatened his career. Once a nurse who was his patient in the Emergency Department wrote a letter describing him as "condescending and arrogant." Another time he had argued with floor nurses about orders that a female chief resident had countermanded. A private patient complained after he woke her at 1 A.M. to conduct a routine admitting physical complete with breast exam.
>
> He was an only child of immigrant parents who had both suffered losses during World War II. His father was heavy-handed, hot-tempered, and argumentative. He described his mother as anxious, hypochondriacal, "a worrier," and "smothering." Because of being eneuretic and encopretic until age 10 years, he saw a counselor who focused on his parents' problems with each other. He had few friends in high school but enjoyed chess, which he continued in college, where he also became interested in science. Romantic relationships lasted only a few months before he lost interest. In the workplace, he was resentful at feeling trapped by women, suspecting that if he tried to defend himself he would be regarded as either controlling or condescending.
>
> A psychiatrist who saw him in consultation noted narcissistic personality traits, difficulty dealing with women, and a lack of empathy. He recommended that the resident return to work after a brief suspension, because he seemed to have grasped that it was prudent to be tactful so as to avoid future damaging incidents. The young resident had also agreed to meet intermittently with a preceptor who could model more constructive ways of dealing with such situations.
>
> At the end of 2 years, he had received no further disciplinary sanctions and ended treatment. However, shortly before completing his residency, he settled a large malpractice suit for neglect of a woman in labor whose monitor showed fetal distress and whose child was born severely damaged.

This resident was committed to achieving the recognition and independence that could allow him to escape his mother's smothering influence—far more than he was committed to empathic caring. He also identified with his heavy-handed father, who, as "hot-tempered" and argumentative, had devalued his mother. As a result, he was confused in disputes with nurses because he could neither understand nor identify with their concerns about sensitive treatment, and he was unable to weigh these appropriately when making treatment decisions. Stuck in Kohlberg's Machiavellian stage of moral reasoning, he had learned to recognize the importance of diplomacy but was unable to appreciate adequately and to be moved by the impact his mistakes had on others. Furthermore, his isolation from his peers and family made it difficult for him to develop the caring virtues he needed to function independently and well as a physician. Had he been less impaired and more capable of remorse, treatment directed at each of these problems might have improved his capacity to feel empathy for and respond appropriately on behalf of his patients.

Obligation

From a moral perspective, people develop a sense of *obligation* to care by integrating compassion into their core commitments. This sense of obligation, often grounded in one's worldview (Colby and Damon 1992), is important in guiding clinicians through the stresses of training and of emergency situations, when patients' needs compete with needed rest and time with family. Many physicians can recall making the choice as exhausted interns whether to sleep or to spend time at 2 A.M. talking with a patient newly admitted from the emergency room. Therapists can cite similar struggles over knowing how to balance the needs of desperate patients with their own needs—for example, for time or privacy.

Principled compassion is also necessary for navigating a course through the turbulent currents of everyday clinical practice—for example, the temptations to be a "rock" instead of a "sieve" at the hospital door, a single-minded researcher, or an ever-more-productive clinician. The greater their awareness of the moral choices posed by these competing demands and of how they are making such choices, the less likely clinicians are to come to resemble the cynical fictional caretakers in Richard Dooling's *Critical Care* or in Samuel Shem's *House of God* and *Mount Misery*.

Cultivating this awareness is ultimately an individual responsibility. However, formal opportunities for discussion, such as participation in the rounds of hospital ethics consultation services, can help both clinicians and trainees learn to assess situations (including their value aspects), identify moral problems, and consider possible courses of action (Doherty 1995; Novack et al. 1997). Some training programs also articulate principles that embody shared ideals of caring, such as "Every patient is your grandmother." Membership in outside religious and altruistic communities can serve a similar reinforcing function.

Nurturance

Clinicians may feel compassion and obligation but have difficulty *nurturing* patients. A few, like Charles Schultz's *Peanuts* character Linus, care abstractly: "I love mankind; it's people I can't stand." Others lack relevant skills and have no opportunity to develop them. Still others feel deeply about certain patients but withdraw emotionally to protect themselves from becoming hurt or spent. For example, after experiencing a patient's death, a medical intern may extend himself less to other dying patients, and a psychiatry resident may distance herself from potentially demanding patients after one has invaded her personal space.

> A 30-year-old laboratory technician complained of feeling that she had never measured up. Her history revealed that she blamed herself for failing to prevent her mother's decline from amyotrophic lateral sclerosis and for competing unsuccessfully with her more sociable twin sister for her father's approval. Obsessively perfectionistic, she tried to compensate by exercising and reading compulsively. Eventually, she lost considerable weight, showed increasing difficulty ending her therapy sessions, and began to call her therapist with seemingly endless questions.
>
> Her therapist attempted first to interpret and then to set limits on her behavior by meeting with her in his waiting area (so that he could leave her) and referring her after-hours calls to his coverage. Eventually when she began walking by his house and her weight fell to dangerous levels, he insisted that she choose between a psychiatric hospitalization and termination of the treatment. He found himself more reluctant to take on patients who might need to call him between sessions.

Many clinicians in training become disappointed in themselves as nurturers either because of having to set strict limits or because they are too fatigued and overworked to care in the way they expected that they would. Their guilt over specific failures to care and shame over believing they are not more caring can cause them to rethink their priorities and reconsider whether they are cut out for clinical work.

These problems at various levels of moral functioning would call for specific approaches: Clinicians who lack a strong basic commitment to caring for others may need encouragement to rethink their career choices. Others whose various commitments are poorly integrated may need to make them more conscious and realistically sustainable. Trainees with difficulty making appropriate decisions about patients' objective and subjective needs may have to examine what factors block this appreciation of what their patients require. Have their original commitments to patients been diluted by other interests such as recognition, power, or financial security? Was their original commitment only a duty imposed from outside, split off from—rather than integrated with—their own deeper feelings?

Those who fail to implement what they *do* understand about what patients need may have to examine their vulnerability to competing priorities (e.g., an addiction to a substance or devotion to research). Those who cannot acknowledge their failures to care may need to be firmly confronted by a person in authority, then provided with support (e.g., in the form of a leave of absence, a course of psychotherapy, or a period of more intensive mentoring) to explore the meaning of these failures, come to terms with them, and change course (Baldwin et al. 1998).

Developing clinicians benefit importantly from inclusion by a nurturing professional community. Realizing that others care for them despite their imperfections can help them recognize and understand their failures in caring, inspire them to care in the same forgiving way for others, and help them bear the pain of losing those for whom they have cared.

More mature clinicians are also sustained by membership in such a community. Among the factors identified by clinicians at a cancer center as important in maintaining their ability to work well were being members of a high-quality team, religious and altruistic beliefs, and the rewards of personally helping patients (Peteet et al. 1989). A nurturing religious community can powerfully foster its members' development of virtues such as hospitality and presence, which link the sick with those who are not (Shuman 1999, p. 142). At my own secular institution, medical interns find it helpful to discuss, in small groups facilitated by faculty, challenges in practicing humanistically, such as dealing with difficult patients, making mistakes, and giving bad news.

Diligence

Providing high-quality care assumes *diligence*. Vigilance for problems in nurturing effectively and taking appropriate corrective measures requires accountability, understood as fiduciary responsibility (Sharpe 2000). Diligence depends on virtues such as conscientiousness, self-scrutiny, and a concern for excellence.

Diligent individual clinicians are alert for depression; preoccupation; distraction by erotic, paternalistic, and other countertransference feelings; competing priorities; and the defensive use of denial. Diligent institutions avoid lax systems of accountability as well as a myopic focus on research, growth, reputation, or the fiscal bottom line (Cassell 2001). Clinical educators resist being distracted by competing priorities such as clinical productivity (Fox et al. 2001).

An academic cancer center with a reputation for having excellent staff was shaken by the deaths of two patients who received massive overdoses of chemotherapy as part of an experimental treatment protocol. Subsequent analysis placed partial blame on the nursing and medical staff members involved, but greater emphasis was given to the hospital's lack of an effective system for monitoring the delivery of medication. The hospital disciplined individual staff members and implemented a computerized order entry system with internal checks. In part because of concerns that the leadership of the hospital might have become distracted by research interests, the hospital trustees also appointed a new president with a mandate to focus on matters of clinical concern including safety. One of his first acts was to rearticulate the institution's mission of providing excellent care along with an environment conducive to research.

In a similar way, psychiatric institutions that perform psychological autopsies have a greater chance of reassessing their procedures in response to suicides.

Both individual and institutional failures of due diligence have led to increasing requirements for documentation and regulation of clinical practice as well as the establishment of oversight committees with responsibility for monitoring compliance. Many of these measures, though onerous, are necessary to protect patients and to help clinicians internalize habits of monitoring, self-correction, and pursuit of excellence in general. However, clinicians also must cultivate the ability to monitor themselves in light of their core commitments.

When a patient with borderline personality disorder complained of increasingly severe migraines, her therapist agreed to give her a small prescription for Valium. However, he neglected to address her parting comment that it was so little as to be "a joke." She subsequently tampered with the prescription to obtain several times that amount.

Her psychiatrist realized that he had preferred to pacify her while protecting himself with a small prescription rather than to confront her feelings of anger and deprivation. He recommitted himself to helping her with the full range of her problematic emotions and behavior as well as to attending more carefully to his own responses.

Conclusion

From the perspective of moral functioning, compassion allows the translation of developing obligations into action. Principles, acquired in large part through identification with principled mentors, provide a basis for making continual moral choices in the face of competing priorities. Implementation of these choices in ways that meet the patient's needs constitutes nurture. Self-correction of failures to nurture and redirection toward virtue results in diligence (Figure 3).

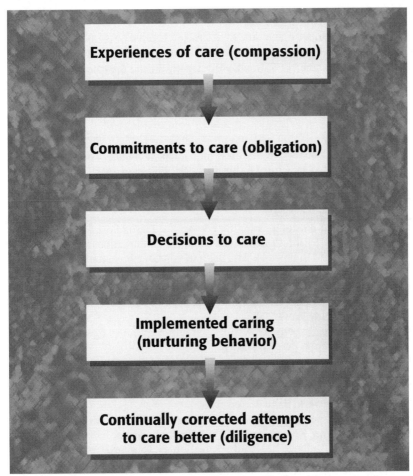

FIGURE 3.   The development of caring as a moral activity.

This moral perspective on caring for patients greatly facilitates assessing the relationship among these dimensions in trainees or colleagues, including whether the aspects of caring are in balance, and why. Does a resident presenting a case to her supervisor show evidence of compassion? Does she feel responsible to act on her concerns for the patient? Does she know how to meet the patient's needs, or does she (for example) mistake comfort for nurture? Can she recognize and correct mistakes? Does she show a balance among these capacities—for example, between following Semrad's injunction to "love your patient" and Bettleheim's caution that "love is not enough"? Does she instead show signs of sentimental overinvolvement, moralism, or a preoccupation with technique or detail? Understanding the moral tasks involved provides a basis for addressing specifically such problems in caring.

References

Andrews LW, Daniels P, Hall AG: Nurse caring behaviors: comparing five tools to define perceptions. Ostomy Wound Manage 42:28–30, 32–34, 36–37, 1996

Baldwin DC, Daugherty SR, Rowley BD: Unethical and unprofessional conduct observed by residents during their first year of training. Acad Med 73: 1195–1200, 1998

Branch WT: The ethics of caring and medical education. Acad Med 75:127–132, 2000

Callahan D: Our need for caring: vulnerability and illness, in The Lost Art of Caring: A Challenge to Health Professionals, Families, Communities and Society. Edited by Cluff LE, Binstock RH. Baltimore, MD, Johns Hopkins University Press, 2001, pp 11–24

Cassell EJ: Doctoring: The Nature of Primary Care Medicine. New York, Oxford University Press, 1997

Cassell EJ: Forces affecting caring by physicians, in The Lost Art of Caring: A Challenge to Health Professionals, Families, Communities and Society. Edited by Cluff LE, Binstock RH. Baltimore, MD, Johns Hopkins University Press, 2001, pp 104–124

Cluff LE, Binstock RH (eds): The Lost Art of Caring: A Challenge to Health Professionals, Families, Communities and Society. Baltimore, MD, Johns Hopkins University Press, 2001

Colby A, Damon W: Some Do Care: Contemporary Lives of Moral Commitment. New York, Free Press, 1992

Crawshaw R, Rogers DE, Pellegrino ED, et al: Patient-physician covenant. JAMA 273:1553, 1995

Doherty WJ: Soul Searching: Why Psychotherapy Must Promote Moral Responsibility. New York, Basic Books, 1995

For our patients, not for profits: a call to action. JAMA 278:1733–1738, 1997

Fox RC, Ludmerer KM: Caring and medical education, in The Lost Art of Caring: A Challenge to Health Professionals, Families, Communities and Society. Edited by Cluff LE, Binstock RH. Baltimore, MD, Johns Hopkins University Press, 2001, pp 125–136

Hojat M, Gonnella JS, Nasca TJ, et al: Physician empathy: definition, components, measurement, and relationship to gender and specialty. Am J Psychiatry 159:1563–1569, 2002

Leape LL: Error in medicine. JAMA 272:1851–1857, 1994

Novack DH, Suchman AL, Clark W, et al: Calibrating the physician: personal awareness and effective patient care. JAMA 278:502–509, 1997

Pellegrino ED, Thomasma CD: Helping and Healing: Religious Commitment in Health Care. Washington, DC, Georgetown University Press, 1997

Peteet JR, Murray-Ross DM, Medeiros C, et al: Job stress and satisfaction among the staff members at a cancer center. Cancer 64:975–982, 1989

Rako S, Mazur H (eds): Semrad: The Heart of a Therapist. New York, Jason Aronson, 1980

Reich WT: Speaking of suffering: a moral account of compassion. Soundings 72:83–108, 1989

Schwartz K: A patient's story. Boston Globe Magazine, July 16, 1995, pp 14–27

Sharpe VA: Behind closed doors: accountability and responsibility in patient care. J Med Philos 25:28–47, 2000

Shuman JJ: The Body of Compassion: Ethics, Medicine and the Church. Boulder, CO, Westview Press, 1999

Spiro H: What is empathy and can it be taught? Ann Intern Med 116:843–846, 1995

Suchman AL, Markakis K, Beckman HB, et al: A model of empathic communication in the medical interview. JAMA 277:678–682, 1997

Watson R, Lea A: The caring dimensions inventory (CDI): content validity, reliability and scaling. J Adv Nurs 25:87–94, 1997

CHAPTER 4

Moral Dilemmas

Being good is a constant struggle. . . . I think that
all of us have from nature a thing called will; I reject the notion of chemical predestination, and I
reject the moral loophole it creates. There is a unity that includes who we are and how we strive to
be good people and how we go to pieces and
how we put ourselves back together again. It includes taking medication and getting electro-
shock and falling in love and worshiping gods
and sciences. . . . We can never escape from
choice itself. One's self lies in the choosing, every
choice every day.

Andrew Solomon,
The Noonday Demon: An Atlas of Depression

Both patients and clinicians struggle to do what is good and right.
Clinicians make moral choices every time they suggest what is best for
a patient or accept a reluctant patient's desire for less than what is best
(Chapter 2). Usually, though, therapists and patients share enough implicit agreement on relevant values to move forward. Moral dilemmas

become particularly troublesome when a patient wants help to make a difficult choice, when the clinician struggles to reconcile conflicting moral values, or when the interests of a third party intrude. This chapter applies a paradigm based on moral functioning to the task of addressing such dilemmas.

Patients' Moral Choices

Patients often bring into treatment their moral concerns about difficult choices, such as whether it is right to get a divorce, how much they should sacrifice for an aging parent, and whether they should expose a parent who abused them as a child. One aspect of a therapist's traditional role is to help a patient clarify the patient's own interests.[1] For example, a therapist might help a patient ask in what ways she would be better off if divorced. Another aspect of the therapist's role is to help patients advocate for the patient's interests when these are threatened, for example, by supporting an abused wife who feels too guilty to stand up for herself in court. These are both implicitly value-laden activities (Chapter 2).

However, patients often need therapists to go beyond uncritical support for their position. They may want help in thinking through what is right or fair. This begins with fully and accurately *evaluating the situation* (Chapter 1). A therapist may see that a father with narcissistic traits lacks the empathy needed to assess accurately the impact of his drinking on his family, or she may help a depressed patient who is giving up on treatment for a serious medical illness to appreciate that his children still care about him.

Other patients need help to see clearly the moral aspects of the issue at stake (Lipson and Lipson 1996). A woman who has been mistreated all her life might fail to see how damaging her husband's behavior is to her.

> A 60-year-old lawyer had grown up trying to moderate the effect of her father's alcoholism on the family, then lived with her mother after he died. Finally, she married a considerably older man, whose critical and controlling attitude she tried to accommodate or escape by involvement in her work. When he was unsupportive during her treatment for breast cancer, she told him that she needed more respect and found her own apartment. However, she felt torn about leaving and continued to spend weekends with him because he seemed so unhappy being alone.

---

[1]This, of course, does not answer the moral question "What is the right thing to do?"—unless one accepts a theory of "moral egoism."

Her therapist tried to help her clarify her hopes and expectations. Was she aiming to satisfy the demands of her husband and her own wishes simultaneously? To achieve the best possible outcome for them both? What were her legitimate interests, and what was reasonable to expect from him? What outcome (e.g., for him to develop some self-reliance and a more respectful relationship with her) could be good for them both?

Patients sometimes need help, as this example suggests, to *consider a full range of possible solutions.* It may never have occurred to a wife who has never done so that she could stand up to her controlling husband.

A 50-year-old engineer who was devoted to his four children struggled with whether to ask for a divorce. He had always found his wife critical and entitled but her insistence that he pay for her parents' vacation home became the last straw. He briefly considered suicide, then asked his therapist if he could be hospitalized, as this seemed the only way to convince her that he was not their "Money Bags."

Therapy helped him examine some of the assumptions that had led to his feeling passive and desperate—for example, that he was helpless and that confronting his wife would destroy her. With help, he began to envision alternative scenarios—for example, leaving with an offer of support that he considered fair, meeting together with a trusted third party, and standing his ground with his lawyer's support.

This patient found it difficult without help to *relate his values to these possible courses of action.* As is often the case, thinking simply about rights and obligations was not an adequate guide to appropriate conduct (Beauchamp and Childress 1989, p. 385). He also needed to draw on his conception of what a good person would do. His therapist considered with him the kind of person he had been. As he thought about the implications of having been a conscientious man whose obligations as a Christian had always given him direction, he gradually came to the conclusion that he should pay for all of their children's college expenses, but not a percentage of his income to his wife, who worked as well.

Many patients look more directly to a religious or spiritual tradition as the ground of their moral values.

A 40-year-old single plumber had been receiving social security disability since undergoing a bone marrow transplantation for lymphoma a year earlier. He had begun to work part time but did not report this income because he was afraid he might lose his disability income before he was again able to work full time. This was a particular concern because he was engaged to marry a single mother and knew that that his disease might recur.

Since becoming a born-again Christian, he had experienced increasing turmoil because he now believed that it was wrong to deceive the government, even to circumvent a law he might consider unfair. Exploration revealed that this growing commitment to integrity competed with a fear (based on painful past experience) that he could never depend on anyone else to come through for him. By identifying this fear, his therapist helped him take its influence into account in his decision making. Because this patient looked to biblical scriptures for guidance, he and the therapist examined how he was interpreting them and agreed that he would consult his pastor.

Cases such as these raise questions that our field has recently begun to address about how clinicians can best coordinate their efforts with those of others who are influential in the patient's moral and spiritual life (Josephson and Peteet 2004; Peteet 1994).

Finally, patients may struggle in therapy with a range of moral questions in the process of *implementing decisions* they have made:

- Am I measuring my own behavior appropriately, or is my self-assessment colored by depression or resentment?
- If I am in fact failing to measure up to my own standards, am I feeling appropriately responsible?
- Am I taking extenuating circumstances into account?
- If I need to accept guilt and take the consequences, am I willing to do so and move on?
- Am I capable of seeking and accepting forgiveness?

A 55-year old gay sculptor asked for help to sort through his concerns about doing the right thing by his son and his partner. He was a self-described "ex-hippie" who had maintained a strong friendship with his ex-wife and their adult daughter. His contact with their 27-year-old son was sporadic, however, because his son tended to be moody, irritable, and unable to stay long in one place. The son's requests to visit invariably arrived with little notice when the patient faced deadlines for work. On his last visit, his son had behaved rudely toward the patient's partner of several years, a man younger than his father, who had tested positive for HIV, abused alcohol, and in recent years had become more emotionally and financially dependent on the patient.

This sharp clash between his son and his partner had made the patient feel guilty and frustrated that he was meeting neither their needs nor his own. He considered selling his home and traveling with his son with no specific agenda other than spending time together (as he did during his hippie days) but was concerned that this might be an ill-conceived and impulsive plan.

In treatment, he began to realize how much trying to please both his son and his lover was costing him. He was tempted to leave both of them but then recalled how important it had always been for him to live with integrity. Rather than taking immediate action, he discussed with his partner curbing his alcohol use and doing more for himself. They agreed to decide in a few months whether it was best for them to continue living together. He made renewed efforts to be with his son when he called in distress and found that his son thanked him for being there. He also decided that if he worked less in order to feel freer, he would still have enough money to retire in the future.

This insightful patient came to the realization that he was looking for a way to help his son and his partner while remaining true to himself. His therapist helped him acknowledge both how and why he had failed when he had acted more impulsively in the past.

Clinicians' Moral Conflicts

Moral dilemmas confront clinicians every day: Should one set a fee that a patient can barely afford? divulge a patient's human immunodeficiency virus status to his partner? agree to treat a neighbor? accept gifts from a pharmaceutical company representative? incorporate one's values regarding homosexuality, abortion, or assisted suicide into a patient's treatment?

Dozens of books and journals are now available to help clinicians think through bioethical dilemmas involving truth telling, confidentiality, competency, involuntary treatment, boundaries, and dual relationships (Preisman et al. 1999). Many of these resources consider how these issues arise in the care of institutionalized, managed care, poorly insured, underage, religious, or psychotic patient populations and in the use of family, group, behavioral, or psychopharmacological treatment modalities (Bloch et al. 1999; Green and Bloch 2001; Rosenbaum 1982). Some examine ethical issues raised by serving in the role of an expert witness (Strasburger et al. 1997). Several (e.g., Lowenthal 2002; Reiser et al. 1987) use case examples to sharpen the questions that psychiatric patients present and to illustrate how principles that are derived from different philosophical (deontological [Kantian] vs. utilitarian, caring vs. justice, autonomy vs. communitarian, rights based, casuistic) (Beauchamp and Childress 1989) or theological traditions might apply (Pellegrino and Thomasma 1996). A few texts focus exclusively on ethical and value issues specific to psychotherapy (Doherty 1995; Koocher and Keith-Spiegel 1998; Lakin 1988; Tjeltveit 1999). Organizations of mental health professionals in various disciplines have codes of ethics that offer their members guidance (e.g., American Psychiatric Association's *Principles of Medical Ethics with Annotations Especially Applicable to Psychiatry* [2001]).

These texts are valuable resources for clarifying principles and for guiding moral reasoning, but what is the process that clinicians actually follow in making moral decisions within the context of psychiatric treatment? What is helpful at each step in this process? Consider the sequence outlined in Chapter 2 (Figure 4).

Evaluating the Situation

Seemingly small details can make a large difference in whether a particular course of action is ethical. For example, the same action by a clinician can be a harmful boundary violation in one case and a harmless boundary crossing in another, depending on the clinical context (Gutheil and Gabbard 1998). Although psychiatrists' training in attending to clinical facts can make them valuable contributors to ethics consultation services (Kornfeld 1997; Lederberg 1997; Powell 1997), they may be less accustomed to assessing relevant value differences.

Asking questions about the patient's and the therapist's values may reveal that they both are committed (implicitly or not) to reasoning on the basis of principles such as utilitarianism, universalism, distributive justice, and personal liberty (Worthey 1997). However, the clinician may need to probe more deeply to learn the basis on which the patient prioritizes or reconciles such principles when they conflict. What is the arbitrating moral authority (Engelhardt 1996; Pellegrino and Thomasma 1996)? Engelhardt points out that for a secular professional, moral authority derives from two sources: the permission granted by each individual and the elements of an ideal world that may be agreed on by "moral strangers"—individuals who do not share a worldview or the values of a particular tradition. Explicit conversations among moral strangers about what constitutes health in an ideal world are rare in mental health settings. Although Bergin (1980) highlighted the ways in which religious and secular values can differ in their implications for psychotherapy, Jensen and Bergin (1988) also documented considerable congruence among the values of mental health professionals. Blazer (1998, p. 215) has suggested several shared assumptions that could serve as a basis for dialogue between, for example, secular and religious clinicians. They include the following:

- Humankind exists in a state of striving for meaning.
- Emotional suffering must be understood from the perspective of the person suffering.
- Emotional suffering occurs within a person's life history.
- Personal histories evolve within the context of relationships.

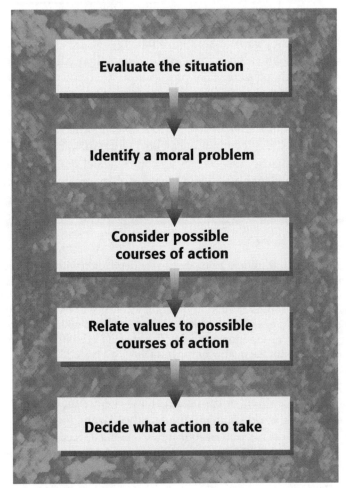

Evaluate the situation

Identify a moral problem

Consider possible courses of action

Relate values to possible courses of action

Decide what action to take

FIGURE 4.   Steps in addressing a moral dilemma.

- The care and cure of the emotionally suffering are shared within a society.
- Theory cannot remain unintegrated with practice in the care of souls.
- Islands of community can be found in the sea of diversity.

Chapter 8 returns to the question of whether assumptions such as these can form the basis for a generic shared clinical morality.

In contrast to moral strangers, "moral friends" share the same tradition and basis for values and can usually agree more easily on what course of action is best. Both moral friends and moral strangers would likely agree on the importance of respecting each individual's religious convictions and therefore with the position of the American Psychiatric Association: that it is unethical to impose one's own religious or antireligious views on a patient. However, a patient and therapist who share a secular worldview might agree (legalities and other palliative options aside) more easily on a choice of physician-assisted suicide in the presence of a terminal illness. Conversely, a patient and therapist who shared the same religious beliefs might agree to draw on that shared spiritual perspective in considering when, for example, abortion could be morally acceptable. Official pronouncements by organizations such as the American Psychiatric Association on controversial questions such as abortion or change for homosexuals may heighten members' sensitivity to the value aspects of these issues by expressing a secular consensus, but they lack the authority that a worldview has to compel commitment.

> A Hindu medical student being treated for depression with medication and a cognitive-behavioral approach asked his therapist about the relevance of his religious faith to his treatment. He reported feeling better after praying and had begun to question whether part of his problem might not be spiritual. Rather than exploring the relationship between his faith and his emotional life, his therapist assured him that they should stick with the treatment program they had undertaken.

Discrepancies between patients' and therapists' values can actually lead to differing perceptions of the issues at stake. Although this therapist saw the problem as one of maintaining a therapeutic focus and appropriate boundaries, his patient felt he was being forced to choose between two paradigms that he feared might not be compatible. Had the therapist considered their value differences when assessing the situation (in the same way he would have allowed for countertransference), he might have been able to address these differences in time to salvage the treatment. For example, he might have recognized his own reluctance to consider a religious approach, then discussed how the patient could make use of the resources of his temple at the same time (Josephson and Peteet 2004).

Identifying a Moral Problem

Identifying a moral problem depends not only on sensitivity to the patient's values but also on a developed vision of optimal care. What are the ultimate goals (Chapter 2)? Consider the example of providing end-of-life care. A psychiatrist who tells his patient that he has a "memory disorder" instead of Alzheimer's disease may be uneasy because he senses a conflict between his duty to do no harm (by taking away the patient's hope) and that of providing informed consent. He may feel that because no effective treatment for Alzheimer's disease exists, this duty is lessened. However, if he is familiar with optimal end-of-life care, he will appreciate that patients with incurable disease often value help in planning how they spend their last days, and he will be aware of data showing that patients with dementia believe they should be told their diagnosis (Wilkinson and Pratt 2002). This perspective is what sharpens his view of the moral issue at stake.

Considering Possible Courses of Action

Clinicians with difficulty considering possible courses of action to resolve seemingly intractable dilemmas may benefit from an ethics consultation.

> With increasing discomfort, a psychiatrist hospitalized a chronically suicidal patient repeatedly over many years. He felt obligated to commit her every time she became suicidal, but these admissions had no apparent lasting benefit. Seeing no alternative, he consulted his local ethics committee, whose members reviewed the care he had provided and agreed that hospitalizations were ineffective. Becoming acquainted with ethical theory regarding futility (that one is not obligated to offer an ineffective or futile intervention) helped him to envision other possible approaches. He discussed with his colleagues on the committee and then with the patient a plan to offer voluntary hospitalization the next time she became suicidal, at the same time reassuring her that this meant no lessening of his commitment to care for her. She felt more respected by his change in approach.

Relating Values to Possible Courses of Action

Relating values to possible courses of action requires the therapist to take her own values and those of the patient into account in moving the treatment forward (Chapter 2). For example, the therapist of the Hindu medical student needed to address the relevance of his own spiritual values and beliefs. Did the patient believe that he should be praying about his emotional life? that he should be praying instead of relying on secular psychotherapeutic approaches? Did the therapist's values and beliefs allow him to support both approaches?

Deciding What Action to Take

Finally, deciding what action to take requires that a clinician overcome characteristic or case-specific difficulties in implementing a course of action. These difficulties could include an obsessional or depressive tendency to hesitate before acting in a way that could be a mistake and to avoid confronting a particular patient because of fear of the patient's or his own anger, perhaps because of countertransference-based wishes to be liked.

> A 50-year-old single office clerk at an insurance company complained of poor memory and insomnia that prevented her returning to work. Exploration revealed that she continued to live with a passive father and a chronically depressed mother, struggled with obesity and compulsive masturbation, and was socially isolated except for limited involvement with a neighbor. On examination she was found to be preoccupied with somatic symptoms and with being prescribed medication so that she could function "like a normal person." Her workup included a sleep study showing mild restless legs syndrome and psychological testing showing depression and low average intelligence, but no other explanation for her memory complaints. Trials of several medications for sleep and depression were only transiently effective. A few days spent in a partial hospital treatment program and months in supportive individual and group therapy increased her social interaction and stabilized her mood, but she felt only a little better, still unable to function as before.
>
> When she asked her psychiatrist to endorse her application for disability, he found himself in a dilemma: To agree that she could not work on the basis of somatization, dysthymia, and passive dependent personality traits risked perpetuating her pathological dependency. On the other hand, she was clearly limited, and it seemed unfair to expect her to do more.
>
> Frustrated with her simplistic insistence on a somatic cure, the psychiatrist was tempted to tell the patient that she had failed diagnostic criteria for disability and needed to at least try to do volunteer work. Discussing these feelings with other members of her team helped him to identify a few smaller steps she could take toward independence while allowing him to better appreciate that she might be unable to take even these steps. He considered declining to support her application for disability, then agreed to support her application for disability if she continued in treatment.

Useful venues for clinicians to increase their awareness and find support for "doing the right thing" include team meetings, ethics rounds, supervision, consultation, and risk-management seminars. By facilitating discussion regarding differences of opinion in difficult cases, these forums can help clinicians first identify with a given position, then examine why they are doing so. They can then sometimes see more clearly how to take their own and their patients' values into account in making hard moral choices.

Dilemmas Involving Third Parties

Clinicians increasingly face dilemmas involving the interests of parties outside the traditional therapeutic dyad of individual patient and therapist. Both spouses have a stake in a couple's treatment. Parents have legitimate concerns about the care of their minor children. Insurance companies have rights to evaluate clinical information in order to reimburse. Organizations such as prisons and the military define the scope of practice for the clinicians they employ. Disability evaluators ask practitioners to perform dual roles by protecting the patient's interests while reporting to outside agencies (Mischoulon 1999). The research agendas of pharmaceutical companies and medical schools compete for academic clinicians' time and attention. Clinicians have duties to warn and to report child or elder abuse.

Should a therapist keep in confidence the concerns of a family member who calls about his patient? What obligations does a clinician have to a patient whose managed care company refuses to authorize further treatment (Sabin 1995; Sabin and Daniels 1994)? Can a clinician treat a patient and simultaneously enroll her in his drug trial?

Consider briefly the process of making moral decisions that involve the interests of third parties.

Evaluating the Situation's Moral Dimension

To evaluate the situation, including its moral dimension, one would want to assess the clinician's primary role. Psychopharmacologist? Family advisor? Expert witness? Loyal employee? Court-mandated treater? Friend? The clinician would also want to understand what expectations and obligations this role entails, and what specific constraints it brings to the treatment. For example, how much consideration of their wishes does a patient's family expect to receive in return for paying the therapist for the patient's treatment?

Identifying a Moral Problem

Identifying a moral problem involves clarifying how the clinician's obligations to patients and third parties conflict. At a minimum, it requires an openness to learn about potential ethical conflicts. For example, a physician might become more sensitive to the inappropriateness of accepting small gifts from pharmaceutical company representatives after hearing how much the industry's marketing adds to the price of medications for her patients (making the clinician complicit in the markup of the price).

What compromises would be required in trying to fulfill the differing roles of consultant, investigator, administrator, responsible clinician, and expert witness (Strasburger et al. 1997)? For example, is the clinician in the role of gatekeeper required to balance quality and efficiency of care (Sabin 1995; Sabin and Daniels 1994)? Does a clinician's accessibility to concerned family members threaten a patient's right to privacy? Is it fair for a managed care company to limit a patient's freedom of choice? What is a clinician's obligation to advocate on behalf of possible future victims of a known abuser?

A therapist treating a patient who had received inappropriate sexual advances from her pastor at church asked if she had reported this to his superiors. The therapist was disappointed to learn that the pastor's supervisor had dismissed the complaint. When a few years later the same therapist treated a second parishioner who reported having been similarly propositioned by the same pastor, she debated whether to tell her patients about each other. Would this be serving their interests, her own, or those of potential future victims? Could she act without violating her patients' privacy? Were there better ways of trying to bring the pastor's behavior to light?

After consulting her professional discipline's ethics committee, she asked her patients if it would matter to them whether they were the only ones affected by the pastor's behavior and, if so, how. Out of consideration for the several parties involved, she decided that if they both indicated that they would appreciate learning about the other and were willing to be contacted, she would put them in touch with each other.

Considering Possible Courses of Action

As the above example suggests, adequately considering possible courses of action frequently requires research and discussion with others. Workshops, hot lines, and reading material now offer information about how providers in other settings deal with the challenges presented by managed care—for example by "gaming (manipulating) the system," learning to use a more behavioral vocabulary, enlisting more community self-help resources, complaining in public ways, or dropping out. Ethics consultation is another avenue for getting assistance in gaining perspective and building options when dealing with difficult ethical questions.

Relating Values to Possible Courses of Action

Relating values to possible courses of action requires clinicians to clarify their own values as well as those of a third party, such as a managed care organization. Such values are likely to include fidelity to the patient's welfare and privacy, informed consent, honesty (e.g., in coding diagnoses or procedures), and protection of quality (e.g., in relation to the threats posed by managed care to psychotherapy). Some clinicians will conclude that they can work with integrity within an organization because they share enough core values, whereas others will find they need to withdraw from insurance contracts, preferring the dilemma of how to be fair to individual patients unable to afford their full fee.

A 30-year-old single unemployed teacher with a history of heavy alcohol use became sleepless and paranoid, believing that he was at the center of a cosmic scheme and might be already dead. He was hospitalized with a diagnosis of alcohol withdrawal versus an acute psychotic episode, then discharged a week later on a regimen of antipsychotic medication. He became sober through Alcoholics Anonymous but discontinued his medication. When he required readmission for increasing psychotic symptoms, his parents urged him to return to live with them in another state. When he refused, they agreed to support his seeing a psychiatrist where he lived.

However, he refused permission for his new psychiatrist to call his parents, emphasizing that his independence was very important to him, that his mother was too intrusive to be trusted, and that he suspected that many people were talking behind his back. As he again discontinued his medication and became progressively disorganized, his mother called and e-mailed his psychiatrist repeatedly. At first, she asked questions about what the psychiatrist thought about her son's condition, then about what he recommended she do. She pleaded with him not to tell her son about these contacts, insisting that it would destroy his trust in both of them.

Although the psychiatrist felt clearly obligated to respect the confidentiality of the content of his sessions with the patient, he was less sure how to resolve his competing responsibilities to the patient and his mother as her son's major support. He tried to achieve an alliance with the patient, but the patient seemed unable to trust him or even to manage his life without considerable external assistance. He considered several options: reporting the mother's calls to the patient, telling him only if he asked, refusing to take calls from the mother, and giving her as much information as he could without actually reporting what her son said. Reflecting on the value he placed on fostering his patient's independence and on being truthful when asked, he told the mother that although he would not volunteer that she had called, he would tell the patient if asked. He recommended that she seek therapy herself but did answer questions about his general approach to alcohol dependence and psychosis.

Eventually while on a visit home, the patient became so convinced that he was dead that he refused to eat and required involuntary hospitalization at a local psychiatric facility. At that point, the psychiatrist shared information about his treatment with that hospital's treatment team, which made application for a longer, court-ordered process of commitment to subsequent outpatient treatment, including medication. The patient and his mother subsequently reconciled.

This case highlights the fact that clinicians may need to take multiple value perspectives into account in honoring the rights and needs of patients and their caretakers. Greater opportunity to discuss these potentially conflicting aims and to hear how other clinicians approach them might have helped the psychiatrist in this case to deal directly with such conflicts before he came to feel trapped by his patient's and the patient's mother's anxious desires for secrecy. With the benefit of discussion with colleagues and/or hindsight, this patient's psychiatrist might have made more explicit at the outset his practice regarding contact with family members.

There are many ways that third parties influence what a clinician decides to actually do. They include fear of economic damage (e.g., if one withdraws from insurance contracts or risks dismissal from a hospital staff) and of the anger of patients' caretakers who are offended by the clinician's position regarding confidentiality.

Conclusion

Making good decisions when confronted by moral dilemmas is more than simply an individual or intellectual activity. It involves clarifying the facts, cultivating sensitivity to ethical conflicts, considering multiple possible courses of action, bringing to bear one's moral commitments, taking into account the values and wisdom of others, attempting consensus where possible, and finding courage to act with integrity.

References

American Psychiatric Association: Principles of Medical Ethics With Annotations Especially Applicable to Psychiatry. Washington, DC, American Psychiatric Association, 2001

Beauchamp TL, Childress JF: Principles of Biomedical Ethics, 3rd Edition. New York, Oxford University Press, 1989

Bergin AE: Psychotherapy and religious values. J Consult Clin Psychol 48:95–105, 1980

Blazer D: Freud vs God: How Psychiatry Lost Its Soul and Christianity Lost Its Mind. Downers Grove, IL, InterVarsity Press, 1998

Bloch S, Chodoff P, Green SA: Psychiatric Ethics, 3rd Edition. Oxford, England, Oxford University Press, 1999

Doherty WJ: Soul Searching: Why Psychotherapy Must Promote Moral Responsibility. New York, Basic Books, 1995

Engelhardt HT: The Foundations of Bioethics. New York, Oxford University Press, 1996

Green SA, Bloch S: Working in a flawed mental health care system: an ethical challenge. Am J Psychiatry 158:1378–1383, 2001

Gutheil TG, Gabbard GO: Misuses and misunderstandings of boundary theory in clinical and regulatory settings. Am J Psychiatry 155:409–414, 1998

Jensen JP, Bergin AE: Mental health values of professional therapists: a national interdisciplinary survey. Professional Psychology Research and Practice 19: 290–297, 1988

Josephson A, Peteet J (eds): Handbook of Spirituality and World View in Clinical Practice. Washington, DC, American Psychiatric Publishing, 2004

Koocher GP, Keith-Spiegel P (eds): Ethics in Psychology: Professional Standards and Cases, 2nd Edition. New York, Oxford University Press, 1998

Kornfeld DS: Clinical ethics: an important role for the consultation-liaison psychiatrist. Psychosomatics 38:307312, 1997

Lakin M: Ethical Issues in the Psychotherapies. New York, Oxford University Press, 1988

Lederberg MS: Making a situational diagnosis: psychiatrists at the interface of psychiatry and ethics in the consultation-liaison setting. Psychosomatics 38:327–338, 1997

Lipson M, Lipson A: Psychotherapy and the ethics of attention. Hastings Cent Rep 26:17–22, 1996

Lowenthal D: Case studies in confidentiality. Journal of Psychiatric Practice 8: 151–159, 2002

Mischoulon D: An approach to the patient seeking psychiatric disability benefits. Acad Psychiatry 23:128–136, 1999

Pellegrino ED, Thomasma DC: The Christian Virtues in Medical Practice. Washington, DC, Georgetown University Press, 1996

Peteet JR: Approaching spiritual problems in psychotherapy: a conceptual framework. J Psychother Pract Res 3:237–245, 1994

Powell T: Consultation-liaison psychiatry and clinical ethics: representative cases. Psychosomatics 38:321–326, 1997

Preisman RC, Steinberg MD, Rummans TA, et al: An annotated bibliography for ethics training in consultation-liaison psychiatry. Psychosomatics 40: 369–379, 1999

Reiser SJ, Bursztajn HJ, Appelbaum P, et al: Divided Staffs, Divided Selves: A Case Approach to Mental Health Ethics. Cambridge, England, Cambridge University Press, 1987

Richards PS, Bergin AE: Handbook of Psychotherapy and Religious Diversity. Washington, DC, American Psychological Association, 2000

Rosenbaum M (ed): Ethics and Values in Psychotherapy: A Guidebook. New York, Free Press, 1982

Sabin J: General hospital psychiatry and the ethics of managed care. Gen Hosp Psychiatry 17:293–298, 1995

Sabin J, Daniels N: Determining "medical necessity" in mental health practice. Hastings Cent Rep 24:5–13, 1994

Strasburger LH, Gutheil T, Brodsky A: On wearing two hats: role conflict in serving as both psychiatrist and expert witness. Am J Psychiatry 154:448–456, 1997

Tjeltveit AC: Ethics and Values in Psychotherapy. London, Routledge, 1999

Wilkinson H, Pratt R: Breaking the news: do patients want to know that they have dementia? Neuropsychiatry Reviews 3:15–16, 2002

Worthey JA: The Ethics of the Ordinary in Healthcare: Concepts and Cases. Chicago, IL, Health Administration Press, 1997, pp 229–237

CHAPTER 5

Unfair Pain

Whoever fights monsters should see to it that in the process he does not become a monster.

Friedrich Nietzsche, Beyond Good and Evil

We have considered moral functioning in general terms as a framework for approaching a mental health clinician's role in a patient's life. Chapter 4 considered in more detail the task of helping patients to make difficult moral choices. This chapter examines the clinician's role in helping patients deal with unfair pain; Chapter 6 focuses on guilt and shame. Clinicians must be aware that, as in dealing with moral dilemmas, their own moral commitments shape their approach to patients struggling with problems related to moral failure.

Unfair pain is a common concern of patients in psychotherapy. Patients may be dealing with emotional neglect by a parent, harsh treatment by a boss, or insensitivity in a spouse. Many struggle with more severe forms: bereavement by a drunk driver, a fatal delay by a physician in diagnosing cancer, or repeated sexual abuse by a sibling. Should a therapist try to help a patient protect herself, accept unfairness, experience outrage, or work with all of these as possibilities? What generalizations are possible about a clinician's most appropriate role?

Common responses to the moral failures of others include questioning, resignation, blaming oneself, assuming the role of victim, feeling superior, retaliating, seeking public justice, contributing to prevention, and forgiving. This chapter outlines how a therapist may work with a patient who is experiencing one or all of these responses in the effort to establish or regain mental health. The task is often complex because it involves the integration of the patient's emotional, moral, and spiritual life.

Questioning

Questioning is an almost universal response to unfair pain: *Why did this happen to me? Did I do something to bring it on?* Profound suffering raises even deeper questions about one's worldview (Herman 1992; Peteet 2001): *Is this my fate in life? Is God testing or trying to teach me something? Does God or fairness even exist?*

A major task for any therapist is to help the patient to put his pain into perspective (Semrad in Rako and Mazur 1980). One way to do this is to take into account emotional factors that influence the patient's search for answers—for example, the influence of acute grief or a tendency to worry.

> A 40-year-old single accountant came for treatment after his mother's death from lymphoma because of his preoccupation with whether she would be alive if he had obtained a second opinion. His therapist reviewed the medical advice he had received, his history of obsessional worry, and the complex, hostile-dependent relationship he had with his mother. Therapy helped him distinguish his grief and guilty feelings from the reality that very little could have been done to prolong her life.

Therapists sometimes must encourage rejection-sensitive individuals to clarify whether and why they are being mistreated. A shy office worker may wonder whether her coworkers are excluding her from invitations to social events, only to find that they believe she is not interested in going with them.

Another way that clinicians can work with questioning patients is to help them reassess their worldview (Peteet 2001). Does the patient believe that God should protect someone who had always tried to treat other people well because she learned this in Sunday School? Has she examined this assumption since childhood? With whose help?

A 35-year-old mother of two felt overwhelmed and angry as her 12-year-old son approached death from leukemia. She described feeling particularly betrayed by God, because after attending a healing service, her son had enjoyed a long remission. Further exploration revealed that she had a history of childhood sexual abuse, had lived with an abusive husband, and had been encouraged by a priest to stay in the marriage. With time she came to see how all of these factors shaped her view of God as an arbitrary, punitive figure who was apt to ambush her if she began to experience hope or freedom.

This patient's therapist referred her for a consultation with a hospital chaplain to consider whether her views about God fit with what her faith taught. He continued to work with her on how her view of God resembled her picture of her father and how it served to perpetuate her acceptance of her husband's abuse.

Resignation

Many individuals feel they have no choice but to accept the cards life has dealt them—even if it means living with the knowledge (for example) that a sibling is shouldering much less of the burden of caring for their ailing parent. They may also believe that accepting unfair burdens and slights is their duty.

A clinician may have to probe this response to learn whether it is genuine and effective. Is the patient reporting resignation while actually showing irritability and covert resentment? Is he actually accepting and generous or feeling forced to bow before an external, poorly integrated standard? Does he show a kind of pseudo-forgiveness—professing to have forgiven without having gone through the process of acknowledging that he was wronged and dealing with his feelings about it?

Blaming Oneself

A subset of patients characteristically respond to suffering by blaming themselves. Clinicians may have to help them avoid overlooking the responsibility that belongs to others. They may need to intervene aggressively when a patient's safety is threatened by ongoing, active abuse—for example, by formulating an emergency plan involving such resources as a hotline, shelter, and restraining order.

An increasingly frail 85-year-old woman was hospitalized after increasingly frequent falls. Despite her need for 24-hour care, her husband would not agree to sleep on the same floor of their house or allow outside help to come in at night. She was afraid of waking him because he

was easily angered and had hit her in the past but believed the only solution to be continuing to be "cautious" in her dealings with him. Because her clinician saw this plan as unsafe, he filed a report mandating
an evaluation by Elder Protective Services.

Assuming the Role of Victim

Some individuals not only blame themselves but also invite mistreatment by being irritable, suspicious, or accusatory. The more self-destructive among survivors of trauma may cut or otherwise hurt themselves;
some feel that they deserve to be punished or even to die. Therapists can
help such patients identify the sources and triggers for these impulses,
modify entrenched habits (e.g., through programs such as dialectical behavior therapy), and reassess their assumptions as understandable but
unrealistic (Stark 1994, pp. 272–277). For example, many patients experiencing suffering unconsciously expect a reward yet openly mistrust
anything good that happens to them. Acknowledging buried feelings
and their destructive consequences can free a patient to consider more
realistic, constructive responses.

> A 30-year-old sexual abuse survivor called her therapist in tears the day
> after terrorist attacks destroyed the World Trade Center. Overwhelmed
> by the burden of evil in the world and feeling guilty for not being able
> to counteract it, she was tempted to cut herself or to take an overdose of
> pills. As her therapist helped her both to understand her feelings and to
> sort through their sources, she began to consider practical ways that she
> could help the immediate victims of these events.

A victim's instinct to give of herself or to turn the other cheek may
sometimes be difficult to distinguish from self-destructive, masochistic
responses. How reflexive versus freely considered is the impulse? Does
it come after, or instead of, experiencing anger or protest? Is it consistent
with the individual's worldview? Is it supported by a caring community or by a sadistic introjected or actual parent?

Feeling Superior

A different response is to consciously take comfort in feeling morally better than one's offender by, for example, "considering the source." Patients
sometimes attempt to enlist the support of their therapists in doing so.

> A 65-year-old widow brought in a distressing exchange of e-mails be-
> tween herself and her daughter-in-law. The patient had asked that other
> family members help defray the cost of maintaining her 90-year-old

mother in an apartment, but her daughter-in-law had instead accused her of not doing enough for her mother because of the tension that had always marked that relationship. The patient asked her therapist for his opinion of the exchange, and whether the daughter-in-law's behavior was characteristic of a narcissistic personality. Declining to make a diagnosis on the basis of the evidence available, the therapist tried instead to help her understand why the interchange had made her feel the way it had and to come up with realistic ways of pursuing her goal of dealing in the best way she could with her mother.

In this case, the patient was hurt because her daughter-in-law's accusation accurately hit its mark—her guilt over her hostility toward her ailing mother. She was also angry because neither her mother nor her daughter-in-law had been recognizing her efforts to help. Instead of supporting her retreat to a position of moral superiority because she had been treated unfairly, her therapist focused on helping her to regain her balance and her focus on her own ideals and goals and strategies for achieving them.

Retaliating

Patients seen in forensic settings have often acted out their wish for revenge. Healthier outpatients more often fantasize retribution.

A science teacher nearing retirement began to hate his newly appointed department chair because of her focus on trivial details of his paperwork, which he attributed to her interest in forcing him to resign. He drank more, became depressed, and developed thoughts of hiring someone to do his boss physical harm. These fantasies were somewhat gratifying but also disturbing, because he saw himself as basically generous and fair.

The patient's therapist found herself walking a narrow path in helping him find some effective form of protest. Doing nothing with his anger seemed to be keeping him passive, depressed, and victimized. On the other hand, retaliating against his boss as unfair, vindictive, and possibly jealous risked harming both of them and perpetuating their feud.

The patient acknowledged having felt similarly angry and helpless toward his alcoholic, controlling father. He recalled dealing with him during adolescence in passive-aggressive ways before he eventually escaped into academic life. Formulating the problem as a challenge to become more constructively active on his own behalf, the therapist encouraged him to discuss his options with his friends and with his teachers' union. The patient felt considerably better after filing a grievance, pursuing mediation, and replying to his boss's verbal barbs with restrained sarcasm of his own.

The therapist's primary goals in this process were to help her patient understand his reaction to his boss's actions and to address specifically his tendency to behave in ways that were inconsistent with his character and values, even when his anger seemed justified. Individuals with a greater propensity to hate (i.e., to show a generalized, unconscious vindictiveness) may benefit from a therapist's help to recognize not only their aggression (Galdson 1987) but also their assumption that they have the right to lash out whenever they are hurt (Stark 1994, pp. 277–279). Some are capable of seeing how the sequence of vengeance, humiliation, violation, and cruelty simply perpetuates evil (Grand 2000; Margalit 2001).

Patients who can see their tendency to retaliate as a problem are amenable to a variety of therapeutic approaches. Validating that a patient did not deserve her parents' abuse and neglect can sometimes help her to let go of the need to abuse them in return. Opportunity to work through disappointments in other ways can help patients shift their focus from revenge to justice or reparation. Cognitive approaches may help to break the cycle of thoughts that lead from a perceived insult to hostile retaliation (Beck 1999).

Seeking Public Justice

Like the science teacher mentioned above, some individuals ultimately deal with being wronged by seeking vindication, punishment, protection, and/or compensation from a court or other established authority. Many feel vindicated simply by having the truth about their suffering heard and officially recognized. There is impressive evidence for this in the recent worldwide phenomenon of truth commissions (Hayner 2001). On the other hand, patients can also use a court system to achieve not justice but the gratification found in continued legal wrangling. Rather than being drawn into supporting one tactic or another, therapists can sometimes help them step back and look at their aims in light of their basic commitments. Are there alternative courses of action that would be more effective? For example, is the potential gain of pursuing a solution through an established grievance process worth the risks? How do they want to view themselves over time? Will legal victory satisfy?

A 40-year-old single woman became depressed after learning that her business partner, whom she considered a friend, had defrauded her of thousands of dollars. She sued him successfully but lost her place in the business and felt overwhelmed by the excuse this gave her family to intensify their criticism of her. Finally, after accepting a job in another city at a company that shared her values, she felt validated for her integrity and expertise, freer of her family's control, and less depressed.

Contributing to Prevention

A more altruistic response to unfairness is taking action (such as filing a malpractice or a class-action suit) intended to prevent similar harm coming to others in the future. In addition to helping patients to clarify their motivations in pursuing legal action, therapists can help them consider other opportunities, such as creating memorial funds or supporting advocacy groups such as Handgun Control, Inc. and Mothers Against Drunk Driving.

An adult survivor of childhood physical and sexual abuse worked as a social worker for an agency that reached out to poor families torn by domestic violence. Embittered by her experiences and at times suicidal, she found it sustaining to provide others the protection that she never had. At the same time, the cases she handled sometimes overwhelmed her, so that balancing her need for distance and her wish to help became a major task in treatment.

Forgiving

Arguably the most demanding and potentially liberating way of dealing with unfair suffering is to forgive. As we saw in Chapter 1, forgiveness is a process that to be genuine takes time, awareness of one's own feelings, and a serious commitment to let a grievance go (Enright and Human Development Study Group 1994; McCullough et al. 2000; Schimmel 2002; Worthington 1998). Therapists can help patients who say they want to forgive decide whether these conditions exist.

An artist in her mid-50s with a history of betrayals both by her mother and by several men in her life came to treatment, saying she hoped that working with a male therapist would help her become more capable of an intimate relationship. She explained, "I feel like I must have a sign on me that reads 'Angry—keep back.'" However, she left treatment after a few visits without being able to say how her new therapist had offended her.

Forgiving offenses real and imagined appears to have been a central task for this patient. Sensing the mistrust that she brought to treatment, the therapist might have usefully made explicit earlier that he would inevitably disappoint.

In addition to modeling acceptance of their own and others' fallibility, therapists can sometimes teach patients that forgiving festering interpersonal wounds may paradoxically be in their own interest. Hope (1987) pointed out three reasons that this may be true:

- Holding onto feelings of resentment can require so much emotional investment that it becomes self-defeating over time.
- The people who are hurt the most by an unforgiving stance tend to be those who are most important in one's life.
- Because the standards one uses to judge others are often those one uses to judge oneself, forgiving others can temper the rigidity of one's self-judgment.

In addition, for the person who believes that forgiving has spiritual significance, it can be a way of actualizing faith.

Couples in treatment may need a therapist to point out that they face a choice between being right and having a relationship. Gordon et al. (2000) pointed out the limitations of both cognitive-behavioral and insight-oriented approaches to couples therapy in dealing with a major interpersonal betrayal such as an affair. They advocated integrating a stage-based model of forgiveness with the more familiar constructs of these two traditional models (Figure 5).

A married couple in their 40s asked for help in salvaging their 15-year relationship. She felt angry and betrayed that at a time when she had been both homeschooling their children and waitressing so that they could afford a house, he had spent several hundred dollars on a hobby. She wondered how he could be so irresponsible and untrustworthy.

Her husband's view was that he had always been overly submissive to her demands and was trying to assert some independence. He felt that she had failed to respect his own work as a night-time store manager, which had been somewhat curtailed by a slowly progressive neurological condition.

Dynamic factors contributed to the disappointment that each felt in the other. His father was passive, and both his parents were quicker to criticize than to praise. As a result, his wife had appealed to him because she seemed motherly and likely to provide him with the encouragement he craved. She, on the other hand, as the daughter of an unpredictable alcoholic father, had always believed that she needed to manage things herself to survive. When she met him, her husband had seemed eager to have her care for him.

Experiencing her concern about money as a criticism of his ability to provide for the family, he had fended off her questions about his spending as attempts to control him. She saw this as passive-aggressive, immature, and untrustworthy.

Their couples therapist tried to help them look at the assumptions underlying these expectations, and specifically at how each tended to misread what was consciously motivating their spouse. He made behavioral recommendations that they clarify facts before assuming the worst of the other person, that the husband find more ways to inform the wife, and that the wife find ways to affirm the husband.

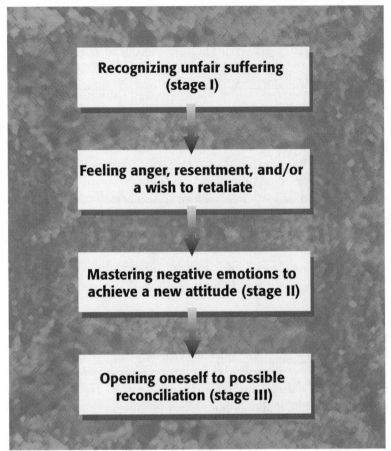

FIGURE 5.   Steps of forgiveness corresponding to the stages of marital therapy of Gordon et al. (2000).

However, both of them felt too wronged, hurt, and mistrustful to try. The therapist explained that to improve their relationship, they would both need to let go of the ways they had related to each other in the past, including the need to be right. Bringing out the impact of the husband's spending on his wife and the impact on him of her accusations that he was irresponsible helped each of them to absorb the impact of these hurts (stage I of the model of forgiveness described by Gordon et al. [2000]). Afterward, they were more able to entertain the therapist's alternative explanations of what these meant (stage II). Considering together possible alternatives to what they feared would happen allowed each to reconsider trusting the other's goodwill. For example, the husband agreed to speak up if he disagreed about money matters, and the wife agreed to ask for his input before taking a firm position about their budget in the future. Feeling respected and affirmed by seeing the other follow through on these promises, they could to begin to move forward on this new basis (stage III).

Without having used the term *forgiveness*, the therapist incorporated its essential elements into his plan for rebuilding this couple's relationship, both by pointing out the need for each to flexibly try again and by making it more possible for each partner to do so.

When patients say, "I know I should forgive, but . . ." therapists can usefully explore both their reservations and their sense of obligation. In a couple, does either patient feel externally imposed on by, for example, a parental or other authority? How integrated are these two urges with the way the patient views the world? A person who sees herself as fallible or sinful and hence in need of forgiveness herself may find it natural to forgive a fellow human being. One who is committed to loving even her enemies may even be able to aim for restorative, as opposed to simply retributive, justice. A recent model of restorative justice can be found in South Africa's Truth and Reconciliation Commission, which managed to rehabilitate truthful wrongdoers and simultaneously satisfy their victims.

On the other hand, patients sometimes understand forgiveness, as taught by their religion, to mean sacrificing their rights or their sense of personal integrity. They may question whether they are expected to forgive immediately or regardless of whether an abuser acknowledges his wrongdoing. Therapists can encourage patients to explore these and other questions within the context of their tradition, to reassess their understanding of its teachings, or both. If they are familiar with the teachings of a patient's particular religious tradition, they can help explore these issues themselves (Richards and Bergin 1997; Schimmel 2002).

Whether or not a therapist directly discusses his own worldview in relation to his patient's, he must remain aware of his own moral commitments in order to avoid countertransference and ethical pitfalls. For example, a therapist's own indignation, disgust, or anger regarding a patient's suffering can distort her clinical judgment: A secular therapist may regard a religious patient's commitment to love her abuser as simply masochistic. A clinician who is overidentified with a patient may demonize the patient's spouse whom he has never met and prematurely recommend that the patient receive custody of their child.

Conclusion

Given this brief look at the many ways in which patients may respond to the moral failures of others, what generalizations are possible about the most appropriate role for a clinician? Although some patients do not seem to want moral input from a therapist, many do benefit from exploring all facets of the issue with a therapist who knows them well and has their best interests at heart. Such a therapist might help a patient see that sacrificing her own interests to an abuser to keep the peace in the short run is likely to help neither of them over the long run. Feeling superior offers comfort but can inhibit moving forward toward one's own best response. Retaliation can seem preferable to remaining a victim, but it runs the real risk of perpetuating a cycle of abuse and of leaving an individual bitterly preoccupied with revenge. The pursuit of justice in a public way as a litigant promises social and moral support but can also leave the victim's condition dependent on that of the abuser, for whom he may continue to carry a burden of hate. Forgiveness can be liberating, but it is a demanding path, both to understand and to accomplish.

References

Beck AT: Prisoners of Hate: The Cognitive Basis of Anger, Hostility, and Violence. New York, HarperCollins, 1999

Enright RD and Human Development Study Group: Piaget on the moral development of forgiveness: identity or reciprocity? Human Development 37: 63–80, 1994

Galdson R: The longest pleasure; a psychoanalytic study of hatred. Int J Psychoanal 68:371–378, 1987

Gordon KC, Baucom DH, Snyder DK: The use of forgiveness in marital therapy, in Forgiveness: Theory, Research and Practice. Edited by McCollough ME, Pargament KI, Thoresan CE. New York, Guilford, 2000, pp 203–227

Grand S: The Reproduction of Evil: A Clinical and Cultural Perspective. Hillsdale, NJ, Analytic Press, 2000

Hayner PB: Unspeakable Truths: Confronting State Terror and Atrocity. New York, Routledge, 2001

Herman JL: Trauma and Recovery. New York, Basic Books, 1992

Hope D: The healing paradox of forgiveness. Psychotherapy 24:240–244, 1987

Margalit A: The Ethics of Memory. Cambridge, MA, Harvard University Press, 2001

McCullough ME, Pargament KI, Thoresen CE (eds): Forgiveness: Theory, Research, and Practice. New York, Guilford, 2000

Peteet JR: Putting suffering into perspective: implications of the patient's world view. J Psychother Pract Res 10:187–192, 2001

Rako S, Mazur H (eds): Semrad: The Heart of a Therapist. New York, Jason Aronson, 1980

Richards PS, Bergin AE: A Spiritual Strategy for Counseling and Psychotherapy. Washington, DC, American Psychological Association, 1997, pp 211–214

Schimmel S: Wounds Not Healed by Time: The Power of Repentance and Forgiveness. Oxford, England, Oxford University Press, 2002

Stark M: Working with Resistance. Northvale, NJ, Jason Aronson, 1994

Worthington EL (ed): Dimensions of Forgiveness: Psychological Research and Theological Perspectives. Radnor, PA, Templeton Foundation Press, 1998

Guilt, Shame, and Moral Failure

I see the right, and I approve it, too,
Condemn the wrong and yet the wrong pursue.

Ovid

Guilt and shame, like pain, signal a need to change course. Because they cut to the core of a person's sense of self, they can also be kept out of conscious awareness, contributing to self-defeating behavior and impeding insight. Clinicians often struggle with how to help patients who are convinced that they have failed morally.

One of their first tasks is to help a patient who feels guilty or ashamed to decide whether these feelings are accurate or distorted. Information about how the patient performs basic moral tasks can shed light on this question (Chapter 1). For example, a clinician may want to consider with a patient whether the standards by which the patient is measuring himself are integrated into his moral commitments over time. Are they consistent with the patient's religious or spiritual worldview? Does he apply the same standards to himself as he does to others? Are these standards realistic in the sense that he has ever been able to meet them? The clinician may also want to consider whether the problem is one of implementation. Is the patient addicted? Does he routinely overestimate his degree of control over himself and situations? Finally, the clinician may want to consider whether problems exist in self-assessment. Can the patient distinguish between the blameworthiness of feelings and actions? Is he reflexively blaming himself for characterological or depressive reasons, in ways that need to become a focus of clinical attention (Chapter 2)? Therapists can help patients in recognizing how these distortions operate, often unconsciously, to their detriment.

What if patients are struggling not to correct distorted self-assessment but instead to deal with real disparities between their values and their behavior? The rest of this chapter considers the role of the therapist in working with patients who deal with such guilt by denial, rationalization, or blame, and with those who are questioning, trying to forgive themselves, or seeking forgiveness.

Denial, Rationalization, and Blame

The human tendency to deny wrongdoing and rationalize to protect ones' self-esteem is universal. Abusers frequently say "I didn't do it," "I don't recall," I didn't mean to," "It's not that serious," or "I was provoked." When should a clinician confront a patient's denial of wrongdoing? She might do so to protect others from future harm, as in the case of batterers referred for treatment. She might also choose confrontation to salvage a patient's judgment from the corrupting influence of denial. For example, a husband allowed to blame his wife for their divorce could become too entrenched in that position to learn from it.

Confronting patients about their responsibilities will seem moralistic unless done in a way that conveys concern for the patient's best interests.

> A 40-year-old hospital administrator with a history of chronic depression and drinking complicated by serious motor vehicle accidents revealed that he had resumed weekend drinking but said that he did not consider it a serious problem. His therapist reminded him that his tendency to rationalize similar budding behavior in the past had had major adverse consequences.

The therapist in this case reminded the patient that it was in his self-interest to live up to his own standards. Having agreed on this, they could then explore the feelings that had led to his last relapse.

Intervening effectively with patients who have already lost control and endangered themselves or others may require external constraints such as court-mandated treatment.

> A 30-year-old mother of four with bipolar disorder and intermittent co-caine abuse saw her therapist only sporadically. When actively using co-caine, she rationalized the loss of control of her spending, her neglect of her children, arrests for driving violations, and indiscriminate sexual behavior as the only ways that she could feel free. After losing custody of her children, she became depressed but was able to make a realistic plan for treatment under court supervision.

In this case, progress became possible only after the patient was forced to face the consequences of her actions. Recognizing the importance of coercion, many treatment programs for sexual offenders refuse to accept voluntary patients.

Group confrontation and support are often important in helping character-disordered individuals take responsibility for their actions. To cite a familiar example, 12-step programs such as Alcoholics Anonymous reinforce honesty in acknowledging one's loss of control, taking "a fearless moral inventory," confessing wrongs to another person, making amends, and working to correct "character defects" (Peteet 1993).

Lacking support, individuals suddenly and publicly confronted with wrongdoing can become suicidal.

> A 58-year-old lawyer engaged in a series of affairs, including with mem-bers of his office staff. In therapy, he justified this by rationalizing that his wife was uninterested in sex. When his colleagues discovered that he had been paying a stripteaser to sleep with him, they arranged a meeting to tell him he would have to leave the practice. He vowed to kill himself if the meeting took place and accepted immediate hospitaliza-tion.

The therapist in this case faced a difficult dilemma. Should he confront his patient's rationalization, at least about how his wrongdoing was putting him at risk, even if it threatened their alliance? Did the patient have a greater need for him to remain someone in whom he could confide without fear of the kind of judgment he felt from others in his life? Any doubts about his actions would have then offered a window for asking deeper questions about his guilt and shame. The therapist's attempts to warn the patient that he risked shameful exposure were unsuccessful in helping him change his behavior, but the concern they showed allowed him to turn to the therapist for help when disaster struck.

Questioning

We considered earlier how therapists can help patients think through whether their guilt is realistic. Patients also sometimes wonder whether they are weighing correctly competing moral obligations—for example, whether it is more important to be fair or caring in a given situation (Chapter 3). They may wonder whether extenuating circumstances bear on their failure. For example, a patient may wonder how responsible he should feel for unintentionally hurting a friend. A patient whose mother "always made excuses for me" may wonder if she is making similar excuses for herself. Patients may wonder what consequences should result from their moral failings and how they can make things right. Is apologizing enough? Do they need to be punished or to atone? How much compensation of another person is fair?

Therapists can often help patients clarify whether the need for punishment that they feel comes from parents, religious teachings or beliefs, or other sources and how they are deciding what punishment fits the crime.

> An abuse survivor became oversedated after taking Percocet for a migraine. Having recently acknowledged in treatment her tendency to escape her feelings by taking too much antianxiety medication, her first response was to feel guilty. She then immediately wondered what her punishment should be and decided that she should deprive herself of opiate pain medication in the future.
>
> Her therapist explored why she framed the problem in this way. Why did she feel a need to suffer for what was at best a miscalculation and at worst a mistake she made when she was in severe pain? Did she expect her therapist to be angry, as her father had been when he hit her for even minor infractions as a child? Did she view punishment as a way of holding herself accountable and being in better control? He also helped her look at whether this was the most effective way to achieve her goal.

Patients sometimes wonder whether they can ever forgive themselves or if a supreme being can forgive them. Finally, they may want to know what a therapist believes is fair or right to have done. Exploring these large questions further is usually the best way to move the patient forward in her moral quest. What is the patient really asking? Does she need to know more about the therapist's values to trust working with him? Would the therapist's answer clearly help in some other way? Why is she insecure about her own judgment? Does she fear disappointing the therapist? Does she hope that the therapist will talk her out of her guilt—that is, inappropriately offer to "forgive" her? Having explored these issues and a referral to someone the patient considers a religious authority, a therapist might in the end choose to answer a direct question about his own views about forgiveness if this seemed likely to meet a legitimate rather than an unhealthy need.

Forgiving Oneself

Forgiving oneself typically requires honesty, compassion, and willingness to move in a new direction. A caring therapist can often help a patient become more honest about his failures and more compassionate toward himself. To help him forgive himself, the therapist may also need to help him change his attitudes or behavior.

> A 50-year-old married Catholic personnel director came out as a gay man and found his own apartment. A few years later, he moved back to help care for his wife, who had became increasingly ill. In treatment he struggled with whether to forgive himself for feeling so resentful of her. On the one hand, he knew that his feelings were in some sense understandable. On the other, he feared letting himself off the hook for being dutiful rather than loving toward her. His therapist considered with him what would make him feel that he was doing the right thing. They agreed that it would help if he could find ways to communicate more openly with his wife, better outlets for his frustration, opportunities to involve others in her care, and activities that they could still enjoy together.

Clinicians treating patients with moral failure due to severe personality disorders often need to help them improve basic emotional communication, intimacy, and interpersonal connectedness. Goldberg (2000) has provided particularly clear examples of how to do this in the role of a therapist for patients who are habitually disrespectful or exploitative of other people.

Seeking Forgiveness

As important as it can be to forgive themselves, many patients recognize that wrongs done to others can be forgiven only by them. How does one repair his relationship with a spouse after an affair (Spring 1996)? How can a parent who neglected her children while abusing drugs find their forgiveness? What if the other person is unwilling to forgive?

> A 55-year-old salesman presented after his wife learned that he had visited a prostitute on a business trip a few years before. He felt guilty at

having betrayed his wife's trust and was interested in both regaining it and in better understanding why he had behaved as he had.

He had been to treatment twice before during the course of their 20-year marriage, the first time after a similar episode with a prostitute. Several sessions at that time explored the impact on him of childhood sexual abuse by his father and led to his father's paying for his treatment. The second period of therapy focused on dealing more effectively with his wife's critical, and at times verbally abusive, treatment of him and their two children.

At the time of his encounter with the prostitute, he had been drinking during an unexpected layover, his mother had recently died, and his mother-in-law was dying that same day in another city. He was able to use these clues to reconstruct his feeling states and identify signals of emotional vulnerability that he could use in the future. His wife said that she approved of these efforts but was unwilling to say that she forgave him unless he and his therapist could guarantee that his behavior would never be repeated. Treatment then returned to the earlier tasks of recognizing when he had done what he reasonably could do and of being as realistic as possible in what he expected of her.

The Catholic personnel director discussed earlier used his therapist almost as he might have used a confessor. To what extent is this a legitimate function of a therapist? What are the limits and potential problems of assuming this role? Without taking on the problematic role of a religious authority, a therapist can often help patients address obstacles that hinder their search for ultimate forgiveness. For example, most religious traditions recognize the importance of being honest (as in confession), experiencing compassion (in this case, God's), and changing both one's heart and behavior (repentance). Clinicians cannot prescribe the radical, transforming repentance that "twice-born" (cf. William James) individuals such as St. Paul, Augustine, Martin Luther, and C.S. Lewis experienced. However, they can and do recommend that patients investigate 12-step programs, which come close, with their emphasis on surrender to a higher power and moral reorientation, including by making amends.

One obstacle that patients commonly encounter in seeking divine forgiveness is disillusionment with a judgmental religious community. For example, certain religious institutions sometimes rebuff the efforts of lapsed members to return because of their divorced status or gay lifestyle. Therapists can sometimes help depressed or abused individuals recognize that they may be hearing religious teaching as more condemning than it really is. They may even be able to help such patients think through whether such teachings accurately represent what a supreme being is like and whether other clergy or faith communities might offer alternative ways back to a God (Ruiz et al. 2002).

The complex task of dealing effectively with distressing moral failures is not always a reasonable goal for a therapist.

An 80-year-old semiretired Jewish salesman with a slowly progressive, painful, and disfiguring illness accepted a psychiatric referral after becoming tearful and ambivalent about continuing to live in pain. Sessions typically began with charming, self-deprecating anecdotes that evoked appreciation for his endearing qualities. He seemed proud of having been a fair, engaging, and self-made businessman, a favorite of his doctors, and a generous father who helped his daughters attend the best schools. However, he also soon revealed that he had been chronically unfaithful to his wife when he had traveled, though he said that he could never tell her this. Although he belonged to a synagogue, he was not actively religious and seemed to have no one else with whom he could review his life and unburden his troubled conscience before he died.

His therapist felt he had helped his patient by listening in an admiring way, but he also wondered whether he might also have inadvertently supported the patient's use of rationalization to justify, rather than seek meaningful forgiveness for, his affairs. He concluded that without enough regret, his patient lacked the motivation to complete the unfinished business he had with himself and with his wife.

Conclusion

Therapists can help patients struggling with guilt and shame in several ways. They can help patients clarify whether these emotions are distorted or realistic and understand their influence on feelings and actions. Therapists can also help patients deal more effectively with realistic guilt. When what patients need most (e.g., moral answers or forgiveness) goes beyond what therapists have to offer, therapists can point them elsewhere.

References

Goldberg C: The Evil We Do: The Psychoanalysis of Destructive People. Amherst, NY, Prometheus Books, 2000

Peteet JR: A closer look at the role of a spiritual approach in addictions treatment. J Subst Abuse Treat 10:263–267, 1993

Ruiz P, Lile B, Matorin AA: Treatment of a dually diagnosed gay male patient: a psychotherapy perspective. Am J Psychiatry 159:209–215, 2002

Spring JA: After the Affair: Healing the Pain and Rebuilding Trust When a Partner Has Been Unfaithful. New York, HarperCollins, 1996

CHAPTER 7

Moral Growth and Transformation

Forgive yourself before you die. Then forgive others.

Morrie Schwartz,
in Mitch Albom's Tuesdays With Morrie

Though much has been written about the moral development of children, moral growth continues into adulthood. We have seen how therapists can help patients develop in their capacities to deal with moral dilemmas, guilt, and unfair suffering. This chapter considers the therapist's role in helping individuals to experience moral growth in other contexts. Clinicians commonly witness such change in patients who are facing death, recovering from addiction, or searching for existential or spiritual direction and may actually find themselves serving as models for demoralized patients looking to identify with an ideal. These situations raise questions about the nature of the clinician's role. What are the appropriate limits of a therapist's involvement? When should the therapist say, "It may be helpful for you to continue this exploration with a spiritual director [priest, rabbi, etc.]"?

Patients Facing Death

The approach of death challenges individuals to reassess their priorities and relationships. Dying well, one hospice expert has pointed out, involves saying five things: *I forgive you, Forgive me, Thank you, I love you,* and *Good-bye* (Byock 1997). Clinicians can often help patients facing death not only to resolve remaining conflicts but also to articulate what other people have meant to them (E. Cassem, personal communication, May 2002).

> A 60-year-old woman with metastatic colon cancer requested psychiatric consultation because of unfinished family business in light of the limited time she had left. She had been a strong-willed writer and activist who had become increasingly uncomfortable having to depend on a local daughter. Her highly successful older daughter had moved away several years before and rarely returned to visit. Neither daughter felt able to confront her mother about the erratic way she had cared for them during their teenage years after their father died.
>
> The psychiatrist facilitated a family meeting at which the patient raised familiar concerns about her daughters' behavior. For the first time, however, she listened while they told her how difficult she had been. In the process of an emotional confrontation, she apologized for having failed them and then told them how proud she was of who they had become. They thanked her for specific ways she had inspired them to achieve, and they agreed to try to care for her in a new way.
>
> Both the patient and her older daughter attended the meeting fearful of seeing old hurts reengage familiar cycles of recrimination. The psychiatrist acknowledged this history but suggested that this safe setting could enable them to have an different experience. Family members responded by beginning to relate in a different way consistent with their highest values.

Individuals Recovering From Addiction

Many individuals who are recovering from addiction experience impressive changes from being self-centered and in denial to being humble, grateful, and concerned about others (Chappel 1992). Participating in a fellowship with people who have undergone similar change and who care often seems to be crucial. In a study of 55 individuals who evidenced rapid and relatively enduring transformations as a result of relatively brief experiences, many of these individuals recalled feeling "completely loved" or "like I was in the hands of a power much greater than myself."[1] The fellowship of Alcoholics Anonymous (AA) helps its members to continue working out the implications of such quantum changes in their basic commitments in several ways: by promoting more realistic steps toward implementation (steps 1–3 and 11), by dealing with failures (steps 4–5 and 10) and damage done to others (steps 8–10), by correcting character defects (steps 6 and 7), and by giving back to others (step 12).

> After his third divorce, a 55-year-old successful but abrasive lawyer saw a psychiatrist because of depression and conflict with his female coworkers. His therapist's diagnosis was that he was a narcissistic character who "did not understand women, only vertical (reporting) structures." Skeptical about the patient's capacity for insight, he focused on supportive treatment of his depression.
>
> Several years later, the lawyer was arrested for drunk driving and forced to attend AA. He found himself surprised at how much he admired the wisdom of the speakers, who also reached out to him after the meetings. Intrigued, he continued to attend and concluded, after a few months, that he had "a problem with self-centeredness." Within a few years, he had acquired a humility and restraint that was noticeable to his friends and was actively helping other alcoholics.

This relatively typical vignette raises a number of questions about the role of a clinician in facilitating such moral changes. Could this patient's psychiatrist have done more than simply witness these changes? For example, could his clinician have usefully focused on his character problem before he was sent by the court to AA? Could the psychiatrist have considered with the patient interventions such as AA or membership in a group whose members were committed to an ideal beyond themselves that might have encouraged the development of needed virtues? Could his own empathy, warmth, and expectations of positive change have made his patient more willing to contemplate such changes (Walters et al. 2001)?

Similar questions arise in treating nonaddicted individuals with prominent sociopathic traits, some of whom show radical changes after religious conversion (e.g., Malcolm X and Charles Colson). Clinicians have begun to incorporate moral principles into the treatment of batterers, using groups that emphasize taking responsibility for one's bad behavior, and in the treatment of self-destructive, impulsive patients through

---

[1]The authors of this study, Miller and C'de Baca (1994), told the stories in their book (Miller and C'de Baca 2001) of several such individuals who had had "quantum change" experiences.

cultivating awareness of impulses rather than acting on them (e.g., using dialectical behavior therapy groups). Yet formally incorporating spiritual approaches, even "nonreligious" ones such as AA, into clinical treatment programs can be problematic, particularly for patients who reject a spiritual worldview (Peteet 1993). Clinicians can sometimes find important common ground with such patients in shared values such as integrity and truthfulness (Gilliam 1998; Tessina 2001) and may encourage the use of secular supports for these such as the program SMART Recovery, based on the philosophy of Albert Ellis.

Patients Struggling to Find Existential or Religious Direction

Many patients struggle in psychotherapy with questions of meaning and direction (Yalom 1980). A focus on consolidating and following their ideals can sometimes be centrally important in helping them find their way.

> A 30-year-old graduate student in education came for treatment after becoming hopelessly behind in her work. She explained that she had become withdrawn and disappointed after her mentors seemed insensitive to the needs of disadvantaged students. Instead of returning to school, she found a job teaching high school dropouts. There, she felt energized by the challenge of engaging the most difficult students but became frustrated by working long hours for a low salary at a time when her friends were establishing their careers and beginning their families.
>
> She had grown up feeling protective of a moderately retarded younger sister. During and after college, she had taken a series of jobs in the developing world before deciding on teaching as a career. In treatment she recognized that her identification with her sister had contributed to her making grandiose and idealistic choices and that she tended to withdraw from rather than confront authority figures (beginning with her solicitous, anxious father). She and her therapist agreed on the goal of finding a realistic and satisfying balance between meeting her own needs and those of others.
>
> To pursue this goal, they explored the ideals that excited her. What aim in life was central to her identity? What sacrifices was she prepared to make in order to live out her passion for stimulating alienated students to think creatively? Thinking through these commitments helped her to identify the kind of teaching job she wanted next, decide whether it was worth finishing her course work, and designate time for her personal life.

Many patients look for direction in life to their spiritual worldview. Religious patients may wonder what a supreme being would want them to do about a bad marriage or about considerably less weighty issues. Therapists can use a range of approaches to such problems (Peteet 1994):

• Acknowledge the problem but limit discussion to its psychological dimension.

• Clarify the spiritual as well as the psychological aspects of the problem, refer the patient to outside resources, and consider working with the patient's religious community or source of spiritual authority.

• Address spiritual as well as emotional aspects of the problem indirectly, using the patient's own spiritual perspective.

• Try to address the problem together directly, using a shared spiritual or religious framework.

A therapist might use any of these approaches to help the patient better integrate his ego ideal with his worldview to yield a more useful direction.

A 40-year-old office worker sought treatment for episodes of discouragement and anxiety that began after her parents' divorce when she was 10. Her father drank heavily and her mother was controlling and critical of her, but the patient devoted herself to caring for both of them until they died. Afterward, she overspent, overate, and became increasingly concerned that she might never find a life partner. As a committed Christian, she had always believed that "it was God's job to find me someone if he wanted me married" and so felt presumptuous taking active steps such as contacting a dating service. Her therapist noted a passivity in relation to God that resembled her submissive stance toward her parents, but it was so embedded in her religious framework that he did not feel he could challenge it directly. Instead, he encouraged her to discuss the issue with her pastor and others in her church whom she respected. Through looking at scriptures with her, they both helped her to see God as caring for her whether or not she found a partner and that God was probably not threatened by her trying to find someone on her own initiative.

This patient's growth in her conception of herself in relationship to God helped free her from the influence of internalized parental objects. Concurrent growth in her spiritual life gave her a clearer sense of her own worth and purpose.

Of the four approaches listed above, using a shared worldview has the greatest potential for a therapist to influence the patient with her own spiritual perspective, raising delicate issues of boundaries, transference, countertransference, and consent. Cases in which therapists'— and patients'—worldviews differ also raise potentially complex clinical and ethical questions. Others have elsewhere addressed these questions, which are beyond the scope of this book (Josephson and Peteet 2004). Whether or not they share the same worldview, clinicians can often work constructively with their patients' moral and spiritual resources. For example, a therapist familiar with a given patient's tradition may be able to help her select resources most appropriate to her needs. These could include practices such as reading, prayer, retreats, small groups, counseling by a religious leader, and spiritual direction. A clinician and a pastoral counselor or spiritual director who are meeting with the same individual sometimes need to clarify their roles. A therapist will typically retain the task of addressing psychological and pathological aspects, but by understanding the pastor's or director's efforts to help the patient move forward in her view of a supreme being (e.g., as more loving or forgiving than she expects), he may also be able to help her better see the implications of these insights for who she is and can become (Griffith and Griffith 2002).

Demoralized Individuals in Search of an Ideal

Many individuals come to treatment demoralized by what they have suffered or by their own failings. They may need help not only to consolidate an ideal self-image (like the graduate student described above) but also to reformulate one that had been shattered. Such patients, if they have lost faith in their family and community, sometimes look to a therapist for hope that goodness still exists and for a way to reconnect with it.

> A 50-year-old schoolteacher came for treatment feeling overwhelmed and "lost." He had always worked two jobs on behalf of his wife of 30 years and their three children and was dismayed to find that after he had a heart attack, she expected him to continue providing her the same level of support. Having managed her chronic criticism in the past by acquiescing, he concluded while recuperating that he was no longer willing to do so. When they argued instead, she called the police and forced him to move out. Discouraged that he was suddenly alone, in poor health, and apparently obligated to continue supporting her, he turned to a therapist for assistance, saying, "I just want to be made whole and right again."
>
> Therapy helped him to recognize how much his identity had depended on trying to please his wife, and that he needed to reformulate it. When his wife demanded further concessions in their divorce proceedings, he reviewed with the therapist possible ways of responding and what each would imply about the kind of person he was. At first, he wondered about returning on her terms and requested direct feedback about whether his strategies for dealing with her were reasonable (e.g., by using an answering machine to screen her harassing calls). Over the next several months, he relied less on his therapist and developed

more confidence that he could (and should) stand up to her in ways that were fair to both of them.

During the period when the patient felt isolated and confused about what to do, his therapist played a key role in facilitating this patient's moral growth. For the most part implicitly, the therapist let him know that he did not deserve the treatment he was receiving, modeled respect for his independence, and represented hope for the possibility of a different future. Put another way, he used the patient's need to identify with him to help him incorporate his moral commitments into a more adequately integrated sense of self.

Conclusion

Clinicians treating patients who are facing death, recovering from addiction, facing life decisions, or recovering from demoralization witness or support moral change more often than they actually bring it about. However, appreciating and understanding this process can alert them to ways in which they can incorporate both transformation and repair into their therapeutic vision. Chapter 8 grounds this vision in a conception of treatment as a fundamentally moral enterprise.

References

Byock I: Dying Well: The Prospect for Growth at the End of Life. New York, Riverhead Books, 1997

Chappel JN: Effective use of Alcoholics Anonymous and Narcotics Anonymous in treating patients. Psychiatric Annals 22:409–418, 1992

Gilliam M: How Alcoholics Anonymous Failed Me: My Personal Journey to Sobriety Through Self-Empowerment. New York, Morrow, 1998

Griffith JL, Griffith ME: Encountering the Sacred in Psychotherapy. New York, Guilford, 2002

Josephson A, Peteet J (eds): Handbook of Spirituality and World View in Clinical Practice. Washington, DC, American Psychiatric Publishing, 2004

Miller WR, C'de Baca J: Quantum change: toward a psychology of transformation, in Can Personality Change? Edited by Heatherton T, Weinberger J. Washington, DC, American Psychological Association, 1994, pp 253–280

Miller WR, C'de Baca J: Quantum Change: When Epiphanies and Sudden Insights Transform Ordinary Lives. New York, Guilford, 2001

Peteet JR: A closer look at the role of a spiritual approach in addictions treatment. J Subst Abuse Treat 10:263–267, 1993

Peteet JR: Approaching spiritual problems in psychotherapy: a conceptual framework. J Psychother Pract Res 3:237–245, 1994

Tessina TB: The Real 13th Step: Discovering Confidence, Self-Reliance, and Independence Beyond the 12-Step Programs, Revised Edition. Franklin Lakes, NJ, New Page Books, 2001

Walters ST, Delaney HD, Rogers KL: Addiction and health: a (not so) new heuristic for change. Journal of Psychology and Christianity 20:240–249, 2001

Yalom ID: Existential Psychotherapy. New York, Basic Books, 1980

CHAPTER

8

From Fragmentation to Integration

There is a precise moment when we reject contradiction. This moment of choice is the lie we will live by. What is dearest to us is often dearer to us than the truth.

Anne Michaels, Fugitive Pieces

In the course of all of it we are learning the fundamental principle that ethics is everything.

E.O. Wilson,
Consilience: The Unity of Knowledge

Clinicians not only treat disease and relieve suffering but also work to prevent illness and promote physical, emotional, and social well-being. Health defined in this way involves wholeness and integration of the person within a larger context.

This chapter reviews the implications of a moral perspective both for promoting healthy functioning and for addressing contradictions in the way mental health professionals practice. It further considers various ways in which clinicians can integrate a moral perspective into mental health practice, teaching, and research, as well as a few pitfalls to avoid.

In Chapter 2, we considered several paradigms for healing. Using each of these has an important moral dimension:

A *biological* paradigm might at first appear simply scientific and value-free. Giving an antipsychotic medication to a schizophrenic patient seems a straightforward, almost technical intervention. Yet moral questions can arise from the use of a biological paradigm (indeed, from the use of any paradigm). For example, does adherence to such a paradigm contribute to a view of the person as a material object rather than a subjective self? How much should marketing efforts by pharmaceutical companies shape our view of the patient? To what extent is a person with a biologically based mental vulnerability responsible for his noncompliance or his substance abuse? Is a biological diathesis a fair basis for legislation mandating parity in insurance coverage? Biological factors must be assessed within a larger social and moral context.

Clinicians use a *developmental* paradigm in helping children achieve maturational milestones, facilitating adaptation in adults ("wooing nature," in Roth's [1987] terms), and assisting individuals facing death to complete life tasks. However, as Vaillant (1977) pointed out, it is impossible to say what is adaptive in life without knowing what is important in living. Deciding what virtues are essential to living fully is a moral question.

In using a *situational* paradigm to help patients adjust to a stressor, clinicians are helping patients to integrate an experience of loss or trauma. Often, this involves helping demoralized patients rebuild shattered assumptions—for example, about whether fairness or goodness exists (Herman 1992; Peteet 2001).

Clinicians use an *intrapsychic* paradigm to address problems created by patients' use of repression, splitting, and distortions of reality to deal with inner conflict. Because individuals repress what is too shameful to bear, dynamic psychotherapy very often involves scrutinizing the functioning of what may be a harsh, punitive superego. Treating superego pathology may also involve helping patients to better integrate their commitments and deal with their failures to live them out. This is because unwanted actions—like unacceptable thoughts and feelings—can lead to inauthenticity, shame, denial, and compartmentalization of the self.[1] As David Mura (1987, p. 4) put it,

> [T]he addict to pornography desires to be blinded, to live in a dream. Any element which questions the illusion that sexuality is all encompassing, the very basis of human activity, must be denied. The addict can become enraged by any evidence, such as an inadvertent microphone, that the people on the screen are actors or less than perfectly tuned sexual beings. On a wider scale, those in the thrall of pornography try to eliminate from their consciousness the world outside pornography, and this includes everything from their family and friends to their business deals or last Sunday's sermon to the political situation in the Middle East. In engaging in such elimination the viewer or reader reduces himself. He becomes stupid.

In addition to proposing techniques for avoiding compulsive repetition such as deconditioning and thought stopping, *cognitive* and *behavioral* paradigms offer strategies for patients with addictions and compulsive behaviors to recognize their mistakes, reframe the nature of their problem, and learn new ways of coping with vulnerability. Mura (1987, p. 22) described the moral nature of an addict's learning to see himself in a new light:

> When such a realization [that the addict is responsible for his own unhappiness] comes, the feelings of remorse and shame are shattering; the addict's façade of self-worth crumbles. What is revealed is a scared child, afraid he will be punished and banished for all he has done wrong, afraid he is unworthy of ever being forgiven or even granted the right of human contact (the addict is grandiose, even in his self-chastising). At first, such feelings can be borne only briefly and then are repressed. Gradually, though, the addict learns to accept responsibility without denying the worth of his self. In this learning, a separation is made between the actions one commits and one's soul. Obviously this process, at least on earth, can never be completed. The addict's history has written itself upon him and cannot be erased. The addict cannot unlearn his compulsions; he merely learns new forms of behavior to cope with the compulsions. The ghosts and words of the past remain.

The moral aspects of employing a *relational* paradigm are relatively obvious. Interpersonal rifts typically owe their existence to a sense of being wronged. As a result, couple and family therapists often find themselves grappling with their patients' expectations of others in the

---

[1] As Havens (1986, p. 377) put it, "[A]n individual can 'lose' himself if he lacks sufficient courage to stand by his values. He then 'sells out.' This is a statement of adult compliance or false personality."

room. They may also have to set and to model expectations of their own regarding respect, honesty, fairness, and the assumption of responsibility for one's actions. Members of a couple considering divorce may need the therapist to help them understand what commitments and behaviors would be required on each of their parts to make reconciliation possible. Each would then face the moral task of deciding whether these are consistent with who he or she is and wants to be.

From a *systems* perspective, the historical and social forces that contribute to industrialization, urbanization, subspecialization, poverty, discrimination, and war are frequently disruptive of healthy relationships. Shared memories of past injustices can perpetuate destructive humiliation and resentment (Margalit 2002). Advocates of improved quality and access to health care may have to confront governmental institutions that perpetuate injustice and fail to correct abuse. As Herbert Mowrer (1967) argued, mental health, individual integrity, and a morally fulfilling community are intimately connected.

Finally, an *existential* paradigm has important moral aspects. The task of reviewing one's life in the face of a serious illness involves reassessing one's commitments and how well these have been lived out (Viederman and Perry 1980). Suffering reflects a tension between the way things are and the way they ought to be (Peteet 2001).

Is our profession sufficiently well integrated to answer the moral questions raised by the uses of these treatment paradigms? Consider what divides mental health professionals in their attempts to make patients whole.

First, psychiatry is split in the way that it delivers care. Well-insured Americans receive very different care from the uninsured. Luhrmann (2000, p. 157) wrote, "Psychiatric illness, like all medical problems but more so, is mired in the ugly realities of the American class structure. That is one reason why psychiatric illness presents our society with moral choices." In part because legislation mandating parity in coverage for medical and psychiatric conditions is in its infancy, individuals seeking care in public and private systems have sharply differing experiences. Patients (also now known as clients or consumers, labels that reflect the value we put on them) who are insured under managed care plans find they are entitled to coverage only for "medically necessary" treatments. Because the need for their clinicians to set and reset behavioral goals threatens to undermine respect for the unity and the complexity of the suffering person (Luhrmann 2000), clinicians increasingly struggle to decide whether they should continue to provide care through organizations that offer highly restricted forms of care or treat only patients who can afford to see them without relying on insurance.

From a moral perspective, in order to deliver care more rationally, clinicians and the society of which they are a part must clarify their commitments to human dignity, honesty, caring, protection of the least well-off, the common good, cost containment, responsibility, and excellence (Dougherty 1996; Nicholas 1994). The American Psychiatric Association's (2003) "A Vision for the Mental Health System" spelled out several of these. The Massachusetts Psychiatric Society recently provided administrators of a shrinking state budget with principles for making decisions about prior authorization of psychotropic medication for Medicaid recipients. As Callahan (2002) pointed out, however, our culture lacks a vocabulary for talking effectively about the ultimate value of human life or for making large-scale judgments about what is good for human beings "in the long run." Agreeing on a process of moral decision making for resolving differences among parties having vested economic or other interests can be an important first step in this process, because having an open procedure that is agreed to be fair will make them more likely to accept the outcome. For example, faculty at McGill University recently achieved broad consensus in deciding what access representatives of pharmaceutical companies should have to psychiatric residents (Rosack 2001). Giving industry, faculty, and residents a voice was an important part of this process.

Second, mental health professionals suffer in other ways from the conceptual splits that afflict our culture at large. C.P. Snow (1959) famously pointed out that ever since the scientific revolution, the Western intellectual world has been divided into two "cultures": one concerned with facts discovered through science, the other with meaning appreciated through the humanities. Psychiatry has long tried to remain grounded both in neuroscience on the one hand and in narrative, existential, and ethical traditions on the other (Stone 1984). However, biologically oriented psychiatrists (who focus on symptoms, illness, and their neurochemical correlates) and psychodynamically oriented psychiatrists (who attend to meaning, context, and adaptation) are thinking about patients differently. Each school offers a vision of health and of what it means to be a good clinician—one warning the profession against becoming "brainless," the other against becoming "mindless" (Luhrmann 2000). McHugh and Slavney's (1983) perspectivist model is more descriptive and fully rounded, but it does not attempt to integrate the perspectives of disease, "dimensions," behavior, and life story that describe the suffering person.

Largely because of this lack of an integrated view of the good, our culture and profession remain unclear about the boundaries that should define diseases and treatments. A growing array of phenomena such as shyness, drug abuse, violence, poor school performance, and child abuse, which previously were dealt with by social, religious, or legal means, are now seen as problems analogous to disease processes (cf. references to an "epidemic" of handgun violence) capable of treatment—if not of cure—by appropriately qualified professionals (Barsky 1988; Chodoff 2002). Many in our therapeutic culture overall (cf. Rieff 1966) and in our profession in particular endorse psychopharmacological as well as psychotherapeutic solutions to these problems. However, questions remain. Should psychiatrists prescribe benzodiazepines or selective serotonin uptake inhibitors for the distress associated with everyday life (Kramer 1993)? What is lost by medicalizing the ways in which we care for people at the end of life? How well does the disease concept apply to violence or gun control? When is it legitimate for mental health professionals' organizations to adopt positions on questions such as homosexuality or abortion?

To address such questions, clinicians must clarify and consolidate their shared moral commitments. Satinover (1994, p. 226) argued for doing this by placing the clinical enterprise within a larger moral and spiritual context:

> In my view, a proper psychoanalysis, and psychiatry, should assume a welcome place at the table of human understanding, not at its head but as a guest. It should recognize in a faith that orients itself toward the moral order the highest expression of human character, whose place at the table it would be abashed to supplant. It should not claim for itself an ability to stand above that faith and "understand" it, thereby turning itself into an ersatz faith; it can, and should, however, help people to clear away the neurotic obstacles that make faith—and hence a moral life—as difficult to achieve as it has of late become for so many.

Atheistic sociobiologists will of course disagree with conservative Christians or Hindus about the origins of morality, the content of the highest values and virtues, and the nature of ultimate forgiveness. However, these differences, if openly acknowledged, need not prevent clinicians who hold one worldview or another from treating the beliefs and commitments of another clinician or patient with respect and interest. Both naturalists and those who believe in an intelligence behind the workings of the universe can also agree on the importance of basic moral tasks in living fully. We considered in Chapter 2 some of the assumptions that Blazer (1998) suggested clinicians holding disparate or conflicting worldviews could be expected to agree on as a basis for a shared, generic morality. Jensen and Bergin's (1988) data confirm considerable consensus among a representative sample of mental health professionals that certain moral commitments and virtues are important for mentally healthy lifestyles and for guiding and evaluating psychotherapy. These included being genuine and honest; having self-control and personal responsibility; being committed in marriage, family, and other relationships; and having orienting values, or "meaningful purposes."

A third source of fragmentation is the split that often exists between clinicians' personal and professional lives. By the example of their behavior, medical school faculty present a "hidden curriculum" that rarely helps students to reconcile or to integrate the humanistic (e.g., existential, religious, or moral) and scientific aspects of their work (Blazer 1998; Wear and Bickel 2000). Freud vigorously challenged the basis of an absolute or objective morality, espoused a strict code of personal and professional morality, yet often related to patients in ways inconsistent with his own teachings on scientific technique (Lynn and Vaillant 1998).

Although authenticity has long been a central concern of novelists, playwrights, and philosophers, clinicians have often rejected as "moralistic" any sort of stricture to act morally (Scheurich 2002). Recently, however, psychologists have taken an interest in moral exemplars (Aikman 1998; Colby and Damon 1992; Kierkegaard 1847/1938), and clinicians have more explicitly embraced moral integrity as a mark of psychological maturity (Doherty 1995; Greifinger 1997).

Given these reasons to more fully integrate a moral paradigm into clinical practice, what are some practical ways of doing so? First, mental health professionals can familiarize themselves with what is already known about moral development (including gender differences) and about modern conceptions of morality that go beyond traditional psychiatric ideas regarding the superego (Chapter 1).

Second, they can join neuroscientists, psychologists, philosophers, linguists, theologians, and social scientists in exploring the many questions that remain about the contribution of moral factors to clinical conditions and the role of morality in mental health treatment:

- What are the biological underpinnings of moral functioning?
- What character traits or virtues contribute to optimal human functioning?
- What roles do spiritual experience, religious beliefs, and conceptual moral systems play in the healthy and in the disturbed moral life (Lakoff 1996)?
- What methods universally apply for dealing with moral failure?
- What is the relationship between guilt and symptoms of posttraumatic stress disorder in veterans of combat (Henning and Frueh 1997)?

- How can we distinguish a personality trait from a state of guilt (Kugler and Jones 1992)?
- Does a moral problem such as a crisis of conscience warrant a V code in DSM (American Psychiatric Association 2000) classification comparable to that recently created for spiritual or religious problems?
- How often do clinical problems present with important moral aspects, and how often are these recognized?
- When do patients want help from their clinicians in dealing with moral issues?
- How can agreement on positive outcomes help clinicians address social problems involving behavior, define health, and pursue the goals of promoting health in the largest sense?
- In times of fiscal distress, what values such as commitment to assertive outpatient care and enhanced community supports should infuse and inspire the closure of antiquated state hospitals?
- How do most clinicians approach moral issues in individual, couples, and group treatment?
- What are the effects of their psychotherapeutic and/or psychopharmacological interventions?
- How can clinicians best avoid pitfalls such as inappropriate use of their moral authority to reinforce pathological shame on the one hand or to undermine legitimate guilt on the other?
- What role does love play in successful treatment?
- How is involvement as a person in the patient's life helpful and when is it wrong?
- How should a physician approach a patient who is requesting assisted suicide, and why?

To facilitate exploration of such questions, psychiatric training could include more practical exposure to other vantage points on the human condition, such as ethology, linguistics, religion, pastoral care, developmental psychology, philosophy, and literature. One possible venue for such broadening exposure is involvement with hospital ethics committees, which draw on the expertise of both humanistic and scientific disciplines to address actual ethical dilemmas. Another is course work focusing on ethical issues arising in clinical practice, taught by clinicians who can discuss their own patients and those of other seminar participants (Lakin 1988). Still another source of multidisciplinary stimulation is literature seminars, because great fiction often stimulates integrative thinking at a distance from the clinical fray (Coles 1998; Wear 1997). Charon et al. (1995, p. 602) have described the way that literature can center the examination of ethical dilemmas squarely in the patient's life:

Like casuistic and phenomenologic approaches to medical ethics, narrative ethics places moral dilemmas within the framework of a patient's culture and biography, allowing physicians to ask such questions as "In the face of this life, what constitutes a good death? . . . Narrative skills can help the clinician to be sensitive to moral questions as they occur, to integrate questions about values and beliefs into the routines of medical care, and to make contact with the conflicts, tragedy, humor, irony, and ambiguity that contribute to each human life.

A third way to integrate a moral paradigm more fully into clinical work is for therapists to develop acceptable ways of eliciting moral issues. One possible model for this is the Outline for Cultural Formulation, which supplements the multiaxial classification put forth in DSM-IV (American Psychiatric Association 1994). With credit to its authors, the following is an adaptation of the outline that focuses on the role of moral issues in clinical formulations:

- **Moral identity of the individual.** What are the individual's core commitments? his moral and spiritual reference groups? For religious converts, there may be value in noting the degree of involvement with both the original value orientation and the current one, as well as the degree of integration or fragmentation of moral values present. What means have patients found helpful in their attempts to integrate moral with other perspectives (e.g., 12-step programs, M. Scott Peck's *The Road Less Traveled*)?
- **Moral functioning.** What are the individual's capacities to identify her own ideals and ideal self-concept, to make and implement moral choices, to deal effectively with moral failure, and to develop morally admirable character traits or virtues?
- **Moral dilemmas in treatment.** What moral decisions does the individual face in treatment? What are the moral and psychological aspects of the problems in need of resolution?
- **Moral explanations of the individual's illness.** It may be useful to identify the following: predominant idioms of distress through which symptoms or the need for social or moral support are communicated (e.g., attitudes toward the symptomatic self as unworthy, guilty, shameful, or wronged; problematic views of others as malignant, unfair, or obligated); the meaning and perceived severity of the individual's symptoms in relation to the norms of the moral reference group; any local moral category used by the individual's family and community to identify the condition (e.g., scrupulosity, depravity, spiritual weakness); the perceived causes or explanatory models that the individual or the reference group use to explain the illness; and cur-

rent preferences for, and past experiences with, professional and popular sources of moral guidance.

- **Moral factors related to psychosocial environment.** What are the moral dimensions of relevant social stressors and available supports affecting functioning? Examples would include changes in the individual's spiritual community and the role of religion and kin networks in providing moral support.
- **Moral elements of the relationship between the individual and the clinician.** What are the differences in values and identifications between the patient and the clinician? What are the problems that these differences may cause in diagnosis and treatment (e.g., difficulties in communicating in a common moral idiom; in eliciting reports of symptoms or understanding their moral significance; in negotiating goals, principles of treatment, or an appropriate relationship or level of intimacy; and in determining whether a behavior is normative or pathological)?
- **Overall moral assessment for diagnosis and care.** The formulation concludes with a discussion of how moral considerations specifically influence comprehensive diagnosis and care. Examples include the need to distinguish and address moral aspects of a troubling dilemma (e.g., that posed by the care of an aging parent), to understand the influence of a disorder in the functioning of conscience, to appreciate the potential significance for a recovering alcoholic of undertaking the fourth of the 12 steps (a "fearless and searching moral inventory"), or for a therapist to articulate a moral stance with a patient who persists in self-destructive behavior.

Fourth, clinicians can become more comfortable talking with patients about these moral issues as they arise in treatment. They can validate the language of moral concern when patients use it spontaneously and ask questions that clarify the moral aspects of the situation, including the effect their behavior has on others. Although many modalities of treatment (medication management, dialectical behavior therapy, psychoanalysis) are not conversations, therapists can engage in conversation about the moral issues they raise before embarking on deeper explorations (Chapter 2). They can help patients struggling with moral dilemmas, unfair suffering, guilt, or attempts to answer Aristotle's question "How can I bring my soul (desires) into a coherent, balanced, harmonious condition so as to achieve real happiness and be just?" (Chapters 4–7). They can also, without explicitly stating their own position, express concern about the moral consequences of the patient's actions (e.g., a person who has tested positive for HIV continuing to engage in unprotected sex with unsuspecting partners), stating clearly when they are unable to support a decision or behavior, explaining this decision on moral grounds, and, if necessary, withdrawing from the case (Goldberg 2000, p. 33). Venues in which to discuss problematic moral aspects of clinical work include supervision, consultations provided by hospital ethics services, or the network forums recently pioneered by family therapists in Minnesota (Doherty 1995).

Finally, mental health professionals can attend more explicitly to the ways that they themselves function morally (Chapter 3). We considered earlier some of the virtues that—in addition to knowledge and expertise—make good therapists, such as caring, courage, prudence, fairness, and respect for individual commitments and community responsibilities (Doherty 1995; Goldberg 1987; Wear et al. 2000). By treating her patients and colleagues with respect, a therapist elicits similar treatment and encourages her patients' own self-respect. Having experienced forgiveness herself, she is better able to recognize the need for it and help her patients to find it for themselves. By showing she can apologize when appropriate, she fosters her patients' ability to acknowledge moral failings. Many clinicians find answers to the problem of personal fragmentation in their religious lives, in 12-step programs, or in other resources that offer the conditions for sustaining virtue. We saw in Chapter 3 how important these resources can be in developing and maintaining the clinician's ability to care.

There are potential pitfalls in focusing on the moral dimensions of clinical work. Because moral issues are often multifaceted and complex, they can distract attention from what has central clinical significance. Because moral convictions tend to be strongly felt, framing an approach in moral terms can make it difficult to admit that one is wrong. Moralism is a perennial hazard. In addition, transference or countertransference can interfere with appropriate uses of a moral paradigm. For example, therapists who feel expected to be moral exemplars can begin to think of themselves as more virtuous or important than they are.

Alertness to the moral dimensions of clinical work can help mental health professionals both avoid these pitfalls and transcend many of the forms of fragmentation that mark the human condition, guided by what is good and right.

References

Aikman D: Great Souls: Six Who Changed the Century. Nashville, TN, Word Publishing, 1998

American Psychiatric Association: Diagnostic and Statistical Manual of Mental Disorders, 4th Edition. Washington, DC, American Psychiatric Association, 1994

American Psychiatric Association: Diagnostic and Statistical Manual of Mental Disorders, 4th Edition, Text Revision. Washington, DC, American Psychiatric Association, 2000

American Psychiatric Association: A Vision for the Mental Health System. 2003. Available at: http://www.psych.org/news_stand/visionreport040303. pdf. Accessed April 5, 2003.

Barsky AJ: The paradox of health. N Engl J Med 318:414–418, 1988

Blazer D: Freud vs God. How Psychiatry Lost Its Soul and Christianity Lost Its Mind. Downers Grove, IL, InterVarsity Press, 1998

Callahan D: Slippery slope: medical technology and the human future. Christian Century 119:30–34, 2002

Charon R, Trautman BJ, Connelly JE, et al: Literature and medicine: contributions to clinical practice. Ann Intern Med 122:599–606, 1995

Chodoff P: The medicalization of the human condition. Psychiatric Services 53:627–628, 2002

Colby A, Damon W: Some Do Care: Contemporary Lives of Moral Commitment. New York, Free Press, 1992

Coles R: The moral education of medical students. Acad Med 73:55–58, 1998

Doherty WJ: Soul Searching: Why Psychotherapy Must Promote Moral Responsibility. New York, Basic Books, 1995

Dougherty CJ: Back to Reform: Values, Markets, and the Health Care System. New York, Oxford University Press, 1996

Goldberg AI: The place of apology in psychoanalysis and psychotherapy. Int Rev Psychoanal 14:409–417, 1987

Goldberg C: The Evil We Do: The Psychoanalysis of Destructive People. Amherst, NY, Prometheus Books, 2000

Greifinger J: On the horizon of authenticity: toward a moral account of psychoanalytic theory, in Soul on the Couch: Spirituality, Religion, and Morality in Contemporary Psychoanalysis. Edited by Spezzano C, Gargiulo GJ. Hillsdale, NJ, Analytic Press, 1997, pp 201–230

Havens L: A theoretical basis for the concepts of self and the authentic self. J Am Psychoanal Assoc 34:363–378, 1986

Henning KR, Frueh BC: Combat guilt and its relationship to PTSD symptoms. J Clin Psychol 53:801–808, 1997

Herman JL: Trauma and Recovery. New York, Basic Books, 1992

Jensen JP, Bergin AE: Mental health values of professional therapists: a national interdisciplinary survey. Professional Psychology Research and Practice 19:290–297, 1988

Kierkegaard S: Purity of Heart Is to Will One Thing (1847). New York, Harper & Brothers, 1938

Kramer PD: Listening to Prozac: A Psychiatrist Explores Antidepressant Drugs and the Remaking of the Self. New York, Viking, 1993

Kugler K, Jones WH: On conceptualizing and assessing guilt. J Pers Soc Psychol 62:318–327, 1992

Lakin M: Ethical Issues in the Psychotherapies. New York, Oxford University Press, 1988

Lakoff G: Moral Politics: What Conservatives Know That Liberals Don't. Chicago, IL, University of Chicago Press, 1996

Luhrmann TM: Of Two Minds: The Growing Disorder in American Psychiatry. New York, Knopf, 2000

Lynn DJ, Vaillant GE: Anonymity, neutrality, and confidentiality in the actual methods of Sigmund Freud: a review of 43 cases, 1907–1939. Am J Psychiatry 155:163–171, 1998

Margalit A: The Ethics of Memory. Cambridge, MA, Harvard University Press, 2002

McHugh PR, Slavney PR: The Perspectives of Psychiatry. Baltimore, MD, Johns Hopkins University Press, 1983

Mowrer OH: Morality and Mental Health. Chicago, IL, Rand-McNally, 1967

Mura D: A Male Grief: Notes on Pornography and Addiction. Minneapolis, MN, Milkweed Editions, 1987

Nicholas MW: The Mystery of Goodness and the Positive Moral Consequences of Psychotherapy. New York, WW Norton, 1994

Peteet JR: Putting suffering into perspective: implications of the patient's world view. J Psychother Pract Res 10:187–192, 2001

Rieff P: The Triumph of the Therapeutic: Uses of Faith After Freud. New York, Harper & Row, 1966

Rosack J: Residency program addresses drug company influence. Psychiatr News 36:6, 2001

Roth S: Psychotherapy: The Art of Wooing Nature. Northvale, NJ, Jason Aronson, 1987

Satinover JB: Psychology and the abolition of meaning. Conn Med 58:221–226, 1994

Scheurich N: Moral attitudes and mental disorders. Hastings Cent Rep 32:14–21, 2002

Snow CP: Two Cultures and the Scientific Revolution. New York, Cambridge University Press, 1959

Stone AA: Law, Psychiatry, and Morality: Essays and Analysis. Washington, DC, American Psychiatric Press, 1984

Vaillant GE: Adaptation to Life. New York, Little, Brown, 1977

Viederman M, Perry SW: Use of a psychodynamic life narrative in the treatment of depression in the physically ill. Gen Hosp Psychiatry 3:177–185, 1980

Wear D: Border crossings in medical education. Pharos Alpha Omega Alpha Honor Med Soc 60:22–26, 1997

Wear D, Bickel J: Educating for Professionalism: Creating a Culture of Humanism in Medical Education. Iowa City, University of Iowa Press, 2000

Index

Page numbers printed in **boldface** *type refer to figures.*

W illoughby Walling, of Brookline, Massachusetts, has been painting for 13 years and became a full-time painter in 1999. Before becoming a painter, Mr. Walling was a high-level government official, fundraiser, and administrator of schools for high school dropouts. In addition to a B.A. from Stanford University, he holds graduate degrees from the Harvard Business School (M.B.A.), Harvard Graduate School of Education (C.A.S.), and Union Theological Seminary (M.Div.).

Primarily a self-taught artist, Mr. Walling has had numerous solo and group shows of his work in New York and Boston. In January 2003, Mr. Walling was an art resident at the Jentel Foundation in Banner, Wyoming.

The artwork used on the cover of this book is a portion of what Mr. Walling refers to as a "web painting":

> As a child, I used to doodle by drawing a series of interconnected shapes that grew to cover the page. The "web paintings" are an offshoot of that activity. A triangle is the key component. . . . Three points connected represent more complex relationships. . . . The interrelationship of triangles becomes a web that is both regular and irregular. The resulting pattern has a flow, everything is interrelated but in a skewed way. . . . The relationship of the web to the background is also of interest. Various shapes and colors emerge . . . to add another dimension to web paintings.

The artist describes his web paintings as, at a minimum, portraying "the interconnectness of all things. There is a pattern, even if irregular, to the web paintings and in my view to life itself."